Contents

Modified Fontan Procedure.
By Gary S. Haas, Hillel Laks, and Jeffrey M. Pearl **111**

Intraoperative Echocardiography: A Practical Approach.
By Bruce P. Mindich and Martin E. Goldman **223**

Aortic and Pulmonary Allografts in Contemporary Cardiac Surgery

Mark F. O'Brien, M.B., B.S., F.R.C.S., F.R.A.C.S.

Cardiac Surgeon-in-Charge, The Prince Charles Hospital, Brisbane, Queensland, Australia

David C. McGiffin, M.B., B.S., F.R.A.C.S.

Staff Cardiac Surgeon, The Prince Charles Hospital, Brisbane, Queensland, Australia

Throughout the history of the quest for the ideal valve replacement device, the allograft valve has been conspicuous largely because of the attractiveness of replacing diseased valves with human valve tissue. Techniques of preservation of human allograft valve tissue have been undergoing continual modification with an associated improvement in valve durability. Consequently, extension of subcoronary allograft aortic valve replacement to aortic root replacement and to valved conduits for reconstruction of complex congenital heart disease can now be considered with some confidence in their durability.

This chapter outlines some important historical highlights of the allograft valve, with particular emphasis on the long-term durability of valves treated by different preparation and storage techniques. The viable cryopreserved allograft valve, its procurement, preservation, and insertion, and the importance of allograft viability will be discussed. Immunologic aspects of allograft valve transfer, mitral valve replacement with allograft aortic valves, pulmonary autografts and allografts, allograft valve conduits, and right ventricular outflow tract reconstruction will also be discussed. Particular reference will be made to the allograft valve experience at The Prince Charles Hospital, Brisbane, Queensland, Australia.

Historical Background

Efforts to produce a durable allograft aortic valve over many years have resulted in continually changing methods of procurement, sterilization, and

Adv Card Surg 1:1–24, 1990

storage. The earliest experimental work in animals was reported in 1952 by Lam et al.,[1] who implanted the allograft aortic valve into the descending aorta of the dog. The earliest clinical implantations of allograft aortic valves in humans were also in the descending aorta, by Murray[2] and Beall and colleagues.[3] A technique of subcoronary implantation of an allograft aortic valve using a single suture technique was described by Duran and Gunning.[4] The first subcoronary implants in humans by Ross[5] and Barratt-Boyes[6] were performed using both fresh and freeze-dried donor valves. Subsequently, a number of other methods were used to sterilize and store the valves, most of which were procured in an unsterile way. These sterilization methods included formaldehyde, chlorhexidine, propriolactone, ethylene oxide, and gamma irradiation and storage using a carbon dioxide freezer at $-70°C$. The characteristic feature common to all these valves was nonviability, the late morphologic picture being one of acellularity with amorphous collagen and degenerating elastin.

Allograft valves sterilized chemically had an unacceptable incidence of late cusp rupture. Barratt-Boyes and colleagues[7] reported a 50% incidence of cusp rupture due to leaflet degeneration at 8 years in chemically treated valves. These methods were discontinued and replaced in 1968 by antibiotic sterilization. There was considerable variability in antibiotic dosage, ranging from excessively high doses to pharmacologic doses, as well as differing exposure times, ranging from 24 hours to several weeks. It became evident that both high-dose antibiotics and prolonged exposure were damaging to the leaflet tissue. However, there was a considerable improvement in durability of valves using these techniques, evidenced by a reduction in late cusp rupture.[7, 8] Currently, there is considerable interest in the cryopreserved viable allograft aortic valve, which offers the possibility of further improvement in valve durability.

The Cryopreserved Allograft Aortic Valve

The matrix of aortic valve leaflets contains fibroblasts that are actively producing collagen for maintenance of valve structure.[9] It is this maintenance of the matrix by constant repair that confers durability on normal aortic valve leaflets. Apart from the normal aortic valve, two obvious examples of viable valves that are able to undergo self-repair and hence retain durability are pulmonary autografts[10] and aortic valves within transplanted hearts.[11] Conversely, nonviable valve leaflet tissue has a history of failure. Glutaraldehyde-fixed xenograft valve leaflets were originally thought to be durable because of irreversible protein bonding, but late degeneration has emerged as a serious long-term problem. Likewise, the nonviable allograft aortic valves sterilized by chemicals or irradiation were characterized by late failure because of their inability to initiate self-repair.

In contrast, cryopreserved allograft aortic valves prepared by the technique in use at The Prince Charles Hospital may retain viability.[11]

Valve leaflet tissue explanted up to almost 10 years after operation has demonstrated viability, determined by the presence of cellularity on histologic examination, by the ability of the leaflet to metabolize glucose, and by the successful culture of leaflet fibroblasts. Viability of the leaflet tissue may be important for allograft valve durability. The distinction between viable and nonviable valves was previously recognized by Angell and colleagues.[12]

Viability is influenced not only by the sterilization and storage methods but also by the time interval from death to procurement and by the duration and method of storage. The viability of freshly procured allograft aortic valves stored in a balanced salt solution, as measured by the proportion of fibroblasts able to metabolize radiolabeled thymidine, decreases with time and by 18 days reduces to 50%.[13] Viability is enhanced by storage in nutrient medium compared with storage in a balanced salt solution.[14, 15] A multivariate analysis has previously demonstrated the association of increasing time from donor death to the processing of the allograft valve with late valve degeneration.[16]

Reoperation for allograft aortic valve incompetence may be undertaken for three reasons: technical problems, endocarditis, or valve leaflet degeneration. Reoperation for leaflet degeneration is one marker of valve durability. At The Prince Charles Hospital, in a series of 231 patients receiving a viable cryopreserved allograft aortic valve, the actuarial freedom from reoperation for allograft aortic valve degeneration was 99% at 10 years. In a series from an earlier era at The Prince Charles Hospital, 124 patients underwent aortic valve replacement with a 4°C refrigerated allograft aortic valve, the great majority of these valves being nonviable. The actuarial freedom from reoperation for degeneration was 88% at 10 years, declining to 62% at 15 years. The P value for the difference between the two curves is .02 (Gehan-Wilcoxon; Fig 1).[117] Two reoperations for leaflet degeneration occurred in the cryopreserved allograft aortic valve group. In both patients, the primary indication for reoperation was xenograft mitral valve degeneration, but allograft aortic valve incompetence was present to a mild degree in one patient and to a moderate degree in the other. At reoperation (one at 5 years and the other at 10.8 years), there was thinning of the leaflets in both valves and a small leaflet perforation in one. Both valves were replaced and were acellular histologically.[18]

The degree of cellularity seen in explanted cryopreserved allograft valve tissue is quite variable. Within the same valve, one leaflet may be acellular and the other two may show definite cellularity. It is common to see explanted leaflets retaining only small scattered islands of fibroblasts.[19]

All tissue valves, whether they be of allograft or xenograft origin, reach a point in time when valve failure, due to degenerative leaflet changes, begins to accelerate and the "shoulder" appears in the actuarial curve for freedom from reoperation for degeneration. This shoulder in the curve has not yet appeared for the cryopreserved allograft aortic valve in The Prince

Charles Hospital experience (see Fig 1). It seems that viability of the valve leaflets at the time of implantation confers enhanced durability, although this viability is not completely retained in all valves.[19] There will be a valve failure curve, the shoulder of which will be shifted further out from implantation by the maintenance of viability by cryopreservation. Even if the goal of lifelong durability of the viable cryopreserved allograft valve is not fully achieved, significant prolongation of the time to valve failure will be worthwhile. In many patients, an allograft valve can be expected to function satisfactorily for the life of the patient.

The origin of the cells seen in explanted allograft aortic valve leaflets has been the source of controversy. It has been suggested that the cells are due to ingrowth of recipient fibroblasts into the leaflet.[20, 21] However, the cells are likely to be donor in origin. Pathologic examination of explanted valve tissue over different time frames at The Prince Charles Hospital has shown a picture of persisting donor cells rather than one of dying donor cells with infiltrating host cells.[11] Kosek and colleagues[22] demonstrated Barr chromatin bodies in persistent cells in female valve leaflets grafted to male recipients. At The Prince Charles Hospital, a cryopreserved allograft aortic valve from a male donor was explanted after 9¼ years from a female recipient because of progressive aortic incompe-

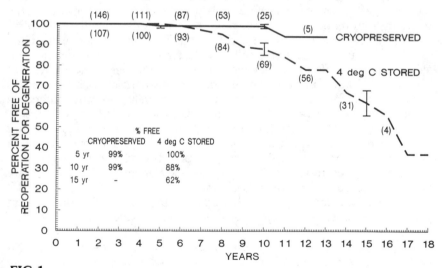

FIG 1.
Percentage of patients free of reoperation for leaflet degeneration after allograft aortic valve replacement using the 4°C stored valve (n = 124, 28 events) and the cryopreserved valve (n = 231, two events). The numbers in parentheses are the patients at risk at each time interval. The S E is indicated at 5, 10, and 15 years. The P value for the difference is 0.02. (From McGiffin DC, O'Brien MF, Stafford EG, et al: Long-term results of the viable cryopreserved allograft aortic valve: Continuing evidence for superior valve durability. *J Card Surg 1988; 3:289–296.* Used by permission.)

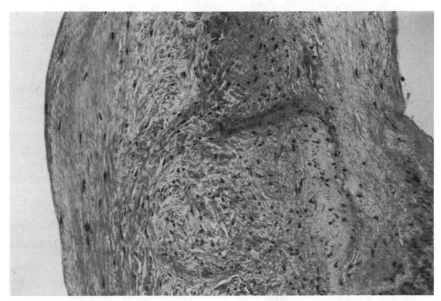

FIG 2.
Viable fibroblasts evident in allograft aortic valve leaflet explanted at 9½ years. Hematoxylin-eosin; ×100.

tence due to a malalignment problem. The leaflets were thickened to a mild degree, but there was no cusp rupture or perforation. Fibroblasts were readily cultured from the leaflets and viable fibroblasts were evident histologically (Fig 2). The cultured fibroblasts contained no Barr bodies, and chromosomal analysis of the cell nuclei showed male chromosomes. A buccal swab from the female recipient showed the usual proportion of cells with Barr bodies. This evidence demonstrates that donor cells were persisting in this leaflet tissue for almost 10 years after implantation.[23]

Additional Aspects of Allograft Aortic Valve Performance

Determination of true thromboembolic events following valve replacement operation is difficult since a number of neurologic events, particularly in the immediate postoperative period, can occur. Such events may be erroneously attributed to thromboemboli from the valve. However, it is widely recognized that, regardless of the method of preservation of allograft aortic valves, thromboembolism is rare and anticoagulation is not required.

Another special feature of the allograft aortic valve is a very low incidence of endocarditis. The actuarial freedom from endocarditis in patients receiving a cryopreserved allograft aortic valve at The Prince

Charles Hospital was 95% at 10 years (Fig 3). The hazard or instantaneous risk of prosthetic valve endocarditis is highest immediately after operation for mechanical valves and xenografts, and this risk falls to a steady level by approximately 6 months.[24] However, the risk of endocarditis where an allograft valve has been used is constant and low from the time of the operation (Fig 4). The risk of endocarditis on a prosthetic valve following valve replacement for native valve endocarditis is considerably increased, and under these circumstances the allograft aortic valve may be the preferable replacement device. The allograft aortic valve is also very useful in the setting of endocarditis where aortic root destruction has occurred.[25]

Allograft valve incompetence of a mild degree is common early after operation and is usually obvious within several weeks. Khanna and colleagues[8] reported a 12% incidence of early mild aortic regurgitation. This regurgitation is usually due to distortion of the valve during its insertion and is rarely progressive.

Significant gradients across the allograft valve are very unusual, even when implanted in the small aortic root,[26] and consequently the allograft offers an alternative to a low-profile mechanical valve or to an aortic root enlargement procedure. In the treatment of aortic valve lesions in children, the allograft valve has significant advantages.

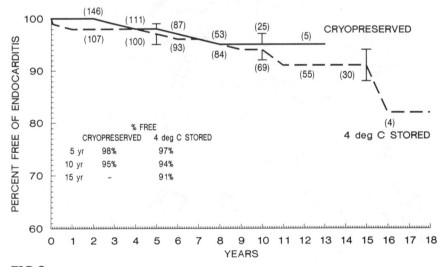

FIG 3.
Percentage of patients free of allograft valve endocarditis for the 4°C stored valve (nine events) and the cryopreserved valve (five events). Vertical axis ranges from 60% to 100%. Presentation is as in Fig 1. The P value for the difference is .23. (From McGiffin DC, O'Brien MF, Stafford EG, et al: Long-term results of viable cryopreserved allograft aortic valve: Continuing evidence for superior valve durability. *J Card Surg 1988;* 3:289–296. Used by permission.)

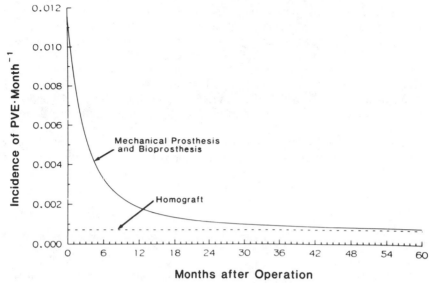

FIG 4.
Hazard function analysis of prosthetic valve endocarditis in 147 patients receiving mechanical prostheses and bioprostheses (1976–1980) and 71 patients receiving an allograft aortic valve (1976–1980). (From Kirklin JW, Barratt-Boyes BG: *Cardiac Surgery: Indications, Techniques and Results.* New York, John Wiley & Sons, 1986. Used by permission.)

Immunologic Aspects of Aortic Allograft Valves

It seems likely from available experimental work that an immunologic response is mounted against the implanted allograft aortic valve. The degree of antigen expression is likely to be determined in part by the viability of the allograft endothelium. However, interpretation of the literature is complicated by the variety of allograft preservation methods and intervals from procurement to storage, both factors that importantly influence viability. Nevertheless, some observations can be made that are relevant to the cryopreserved allograft aortic valve.

It appears that valve leaflet tissue is antigenic, as determined by experiments using inbred strains of rats[27] and human valve tissue.[28] This contrasts with earlier work[29] using inbred rats that indicated that aortic valve immunogenicity was due primarily to the rim of myocardial tissue accompanying the valve tissue and that the leaflet tissue itself was not antigenic. Recently, Yacoub and colleagues[30] have demonstrated class I antigens (against which the cellular limb of the immune response is directed) and class II antigens (required for antigen presentation to the immune system) in human leaflet tissue using monoclonal antibodies. Class I positivity was found in the endothelium as well as in the matrix of the leaflet, associated with leukocytes. Class II positivity was found only in the matrix, most likely associated with dendritic cells. This valve material was obtained at autopsy and from cardiac transplant recipients, and the antigen positivity could not be detected after antibiotic sterilization or storage in medium for 48 hours. However, Yankah and colleagues[28] demonstrated both class I and II antigens on the endothelial cells of viable cryopreserved allografts after 12 weeks of storage. Allograft leaflet tissue preserved for 5 days at 4°C had no viable endothelial cells, and no class I or II antigens could be demonstrated.

As mentioned, the important corollary to the observation that allograft valve leaflets are antigenic is that this antigenicity depends on viability of the leaflet endothelial cells. Consequently, all of these data must be interpreted in the light of sterilization and storage techniques, which influence endothelial cell viability.

It is likely that leaflet tissue is less antigenic than myocardial muscle, skin, or kidney.[29] Some of the conflict among the results of experimental work investigating leaflet tissue antigen expression may partly reflect lower antigenicity of this tissue.

An important observation that can be made is that allograft leaflet tissue with viable endothelial cells does undergo a rejection response. Early experimental work by Mohri and colleagues[31] implied that allograft valve tissue had low antigenicity. They suggested that the subcoronary position for implantation of the allograft valve was an immunologically privileged site because of the finding in dogs of an immune reaction to subcutaneously implanted valve leaflets and a lack of accelerated rejection of a subcoronary allograft valve despite prior sensitization with a donor skin graft and a concurrent second-set skin graft rejection with a further skin graft.

However, Yankah and colleagues,[32] using the inbred rat model, demonstrated that an immunologic response occurs against the allograft valve. Leaflet endothelial cells were lost owing to rejection, with the immune response being demonstrated by accelerated rejection of skin grafts from the valve donor strain and by the generation of specific antidonor antibodies. The strength of the response was directly related to the degree of histoincompatibility of the donor and recipient strains. In this model, muscle attached to the aortic anulus was also transplanted, and this could have been the major source of antigens for sensitization. However, in the inbred rat model of Thiede and associates,[27] only aortic allograft leaflet tissue was transplanted into the recipient's abdominal aorta. They demonstrated that leaflet tissue itself was able to sensitize the recipient.

In the weakly allogeneic system, cell-mediated reactivity by donor-specific skin transplants was demonstrated, but in the strongly allogeneic donor-recipient combination, both cell-mediated and humorally mediated reactivity were demonstrated. Because of this immune response, it has been suggested that ensuring histocompatibility in the clinical situation may be advisable.[32] No relationship has been found between ABO and rhesus blood group mismatch between donor and recipient and subsequent valve durability.[23] This fact was also demonstrated in another series,[33] but the valves were sterilized by irradiation and almost certainly were nonviable. The use of low-dose immunosuppression in the first few weeks after allograft valve implantation has been advised[32] and also used clinically.[34] However, with the low probability of early and late valve failure due to degenerative changes of the cryopreserved allograft valve in The Prince Charles Hospital experience, the possible advantages of short-term, low-dose immunosuppression and donor-recipient histocompatibility may not be significant.

The current data indicate that an immunologic response does occur against viable allograft valves, but from a clinical standpoint, its importance is uncertain and may not be too significant for the long-term function of the allograft valve.

Method of Procurement and Preservation of Allograft Aortic Valves

From 1969 to 1985, the only source of allograft aortic valves was from coroners' autopsies, but more recently allograft valves have been procured as well from organ donors at the time of organ harvesting. All donors must be less than 55 years of age, with no evidence of malignant neoplasia or systemic infection. Procurement must occur within 24 hours of cessation of the circulation. The shortest time interval from death to procurement is desirable, and at The Prince Charles Hospital, the mean interval has been under 15 hours. The ability of the valve tissue to synthesize protein, reflecting viability, is markedly reduced after 24 hours at normal temperature.[35] Furthermore, valves stored at 4°C and obtained 20 to 30 hours postmortem have a markedly reduced proportion of viable endothelial cells.[36] There is a suggestion that antibiotic-sterilized allograft aortic valves may have a higher incidence of postoperative aortic incompetence where valves were procured from donors older than 45 years.[8]

A number of donor details are recorded at the time of valve procurement: a donor identification number, age, sex, cause of death, and time from death until valve collection. A blood sample is obtained for blood grouping, for human immunodeficiency virus and hepatitis serologic testing, and for bacterial culture. Cytomegalovirus serologic testing is performed on blood from infant donors. Donor identification details are recorded, but confidentiality is maintained.

The heart, including the pulmonary bifurcation and aortic arch, is either removed under the usual sterile operating room conditions for organ donors or removed as aseptically as possible in the autopsy room. The ventricular mass is transected, leaving the base of the heart attached to the great arteries. The tissue is then placed in nutrient medium (medium 199—cell culture medium, Commonwealth Serum Laboratories, Melbourne,

Australia) containing antibiotics* and brought immediately to The Prince Charles Hospital. Where procurement has occurred in a remote center, the valve and donor kidneys are packed in ice and rapidly transported.

Within 2 to 3 hours of procurement, the aortic and pulmonary valves are then separated and trimmed of excess tissue. The aortic valve anular diameter is measured by a graduated Teflon cone, and this should be the only occasion that a foreign object touches the leaflets. More recently, caliper measurement of the valve anulus has replaced the use of the cone, avoiding surface damage to the leaflets. Following dissection, each valve is rinsed in 100 ml of sterile M199 (without antibiotics) to remove any blood.

The leaflet of the tricuspid valve is cut into three pieces. One piece is placed in a bottle of M199 with antibiotics, and viability of the allograft valves is inferred from the demonstration of a positive cell culture from this tissue subsequently. Each other piece of tricuspid valve is cryopreserved with the aortic and pulmonary valves.

Following a period of experimental work to develop a method of leaflet viability testing, a cryopreservation valve bank was established at The Prince Charles Hospital. Beginning in 1975, all allografts were cryopreserved after 24 hours of incubation at 37°C in nutrient medium and antibiotics. This protocol was continued until 1988. From April 1988, some important changes were made to enhance valve leaflet viability. These changes were (1) removing amphotericin B from the antibiotic mixture, (2) reducing the antibiotic incubation phase from 24 to 6 hours for valves obtained at autopsy, and (3) eliminating the antibiotic incubation phase of the valve collected from the organ donor in the operating room and cryopreserving it immediately after dissection. Cryopreservation of the valve obtained at autopsy now takes place within 23 to 24 hours of donor death, compared with an average of 39 hours before the changes were initiated. Cryopreservation of the organ donor–derived valve occurs from 3 to 4 hours after donor death depending on transport time (previously 26 hours).

At the time of harvesting of valves at autopsy, two swabs are taken from the pericardium and a piece of myocardium for microbiological culture. Following valve dissection, the aortic and pulmonary valves are each placed in 100 ml of M199 with antibiotics along with a piece of the tricuspid leaflet of the valve and a piece of tissue trimmings. The valves are then incubated for 6 hours at 37°C. A third piece of tricuspid valve leaflet is placed in a bottle of M199 with antibiotics and viability assessed by tissue culture. After incubation, the valves are cryopreserved in a manner identical to valves obtained from an organ donor. The tissue trimmings that were incubated with the aortic and pulmonary valves, the incubation solutions, and the freezing solutions are all microbiologically cultured.

For valves obtained in an operating room, 10 ml of 10% dimethyl sulfoxide (DMSO) is added to 90 ml of cold, fresh M199 without antibiotics

---

*Antibiotics include 50 IU/ml of penicillin, 50 µg/ml of streptomycin, and 10 µg/ml of amphotericin B. Since April 1988, amphotericin B has been omitted from the solution.

successfully managed by allograft aortic root replacement, so that abscess cavities are excluded from the circulation.[42]

Allograft aortic root replacement has been used for the relief of tunnel aortic stenosis.[41] Clarke[46] reported a technique performed in three patients that may result in more complete relief of the obstruction by combining the Konno aortoventriculoplasty technique with aortic root replacement, using the anterior leaflet of the mitral valve of the graft to patch the ventricular septum to relieve the subvalvar obstruction. Redundant graft aortic wall is then used to patch the right ventricular outflow tract.

The Allograft Aortic Valve for Mitral Valve Replacement

The use of the allograft aortic valve for mitral valve replacement has been limited and largely unsuccessful.[47-49] Stented allograft aortic valves provided satisfactory short-term results, but long-term results were poor owing to a high incidence of reoperation, as a result of leaflet degeneration, and tearing of the allograft from the rigid stent. The tissue degeneration was likely to be due to preservation techniques that resulted in nonviable valves. The long-term results of mitral valve replacement using an unstented aortic allograft have been reported by Mankad and colleagues.[50] The technique involved fixing an antibiotic sterilized aortic allograft inside a Dacron tube and suturing the tube within the left atrium so that there was a smooth flow of blood from the pulmonary veins into the valve tube. The incidence of technical failure was low, occurring in 1.6% of patients. The late allograft valve degeneration mirrored that seen in similarly prepared, largely nonviable aortic valve allografts. With the development of flexible stents used in xenograft valves, improved methods of fixation of tissue to stents, and cryopreservation techniques producing durable viable valve tissue, the place of allograft mitral valve replacement may need to be reconsidered.

Autologous Pulmonary Valve for Aortic Valve Replacement

Aortic valve replacement using the autologous pulmonary valve was pioneered by Ross and has given excellent long-term results.[51, 52] Despite these results, the operation is not widely used.

Robles and colleagues[51] published the results of 202 autologous pulmonary valves transplanted into the aortic position between 1967 and 1982, with a follow-up period up to 14 years. This technique was used for young patients in whom a long life span was anticipated. The mean patient age was 31.2 years, with a range of 9 to 60 years. The overall mortality was 7.9% (70% confidence limits, 5.9% to 10.4%), most of these being hospital deaths occurring in the first 5 years of the experience. Late valve failure was caused by technical error at the time of insertion and by infective endocarditis. After 14 years of follow-up, the actuarial freedom from aortic incompetence due to technical error was 93% and the actuarial freedom from endocarditis was 96%. No patient developed valve leaflet degeneration or macroscopic or microscopic calcification. Explanted valve leaflet tissue was demonstrated to have excellent viability.

The operation involves the careful excision of the pulmonary valve with a cuff of ventricular muscle and main pulmonary artery. Following excision of the aortic valve, the pulmonary autograft is then implanted in the subcoronary position. The right ventricular outflow is then reconstructed with either an allograft pulmonary or aortic valve.

The good long-term results reported with this procedure are likely due to the excellent maintenance of viability because of the immediate implantation and absence of valve leaflet damage by antibiotic sterilization and also the absence of an immune response. However, when these results are compared with those of the cryopreserved viable allograft valve, the benefits seem to be outweighed by the magnitude of the procedure.

Aortic Valve Replacement by an Allograft Pulmonary Valve

Principally because of the shortage of allograft aortic valves, 16 allograft pulmonary valves have been used in the aortic position at The Prince Charles Hospital. This experience is quite small, with only short follow up, and some valves have become incompetent. Three reoperations for early structural degeneration have necessitated discontinuance of the use of these valves for aortic valve replacement.

Allograft Valve Conduits and Right Ventricular Outflow Tract Reconstruction

Ross and Somerville[53] in 1966 reported the correction of pulmonary atresia employing an antibiotic sterilized aortic allograft as a conduit. Subsequently, allograft conduits prepared by irradiation had a high incidence of calcification and degeneration.[54, 55] Unfortunately, the same problems were encountered with the glutaraldehyde-treated porcine valved conduits.[55, 56] However, a number of centers continued using the aortic allograft valve, either antibiotic sterilized or cryopreserved, as a conduit,[57, 58] avoiding the high incidence of degeneration that chemically and irradiated sterilized valves developed. In the experience of Fontan and colleagues,[57] none of the 68 patients surviving conduit placement for complex congenital heart disease required reoperation during a mean follow-up period of approximately 4 years (range, 1 month to 15 years) for allograft valve degeneration.

Conduits may be placed, as originally used by Ross and Somerville,[53] using the aortic valve, ascending aorta, and anterior leaflet of the mitral valve, or by suturing the base of the allograft to a preclotted woven Dacron tube, suturing the allograft ascending aorta to the pulmonary artery and the Dacron tube to the systemic venous ventricle.

The very low incidence of valve-related complications following aortic valve replacement with the cryopreserved allograft aortic valve, together with the already promising early results of the allograft aortic valve conduit from the more recent era, suggests that this technique will be superior to other currently available conduits.

Kay and colleagues[59] have suggested that the allograft pulmonary valve may be preferable to the aortic valve used as a conduit and reported its use in a small number of patients. They indicated that the larger pulmonary valve diameter, thinner pulmonary artery walls, which may be more suitable to the low-pressure pulmonary system, and better availability compared with the allograft aortic valve may make the pulmonary valve more suitable. Allograft pulmonary or aortic valves may also be used in a variety of ways to create a valved connection between the right ventricle and pulmonary artery by using the allograft as a pulmonary valve replacement in the orthotopic position.

Conclusion

Conceptually, the pulmonary autograft is probably the closest to the perfect replacement device for the aortic valve since it carries its full complement of leaflet endothelium and fibroblasts capable of maintaining leaflet structure by self-repair. However, it is an operation that is unlikely to be used widely since it converts a single valve replacement into a double valve replacement procedure. Nevertheless, the concept of maintenance of valve leaflet viability is an attractive one, and the current interest in cryo preservation and the viable allograft valve reflects this.

The viable cryopreserved allograft aortic valve appears to offer improved durability over other forms of allograft valve preservation. However, it still remains to be seen if this technique confers lifelong valve durability in the majority of patients by delaying the time to leaflet degeneration. This focus on valve leaflet viability, the fate of leaflet matrix fibroblasts following implantation, and valve durability is likely to continue for some time.

What is apparent is that allograft aortic and allograft and autologous pulmonary valves are very versatile and flexible devices for a number of complex cardiac surgical conditions, such as aortic root infection, complex aortic root pathology, and congenital heart disease. The advantages of these valves in certain patients (children, women of childbearing age, young adults, and patients in whom anticoagulation is contraindicated) are so significant that their use should be an important part of the repertoire of all cardiac surgeons.

References

1. Lam CR, Aram HH, Munnell ER: An experimental study of aortic valve homografts. *Surg Gynecol Obstet* 1952; 94:129–135.

2. Murray G: Homologous aortic-valve-segment transplants as surgical treatment for aortic and mitral insufficiency. *Angiology* 1956; 7:466–471.
3. Beall AC, Morris GC, Cooley DA, et al: Homotransplantation of the aortic valve. *J Thorac Cardiovasc Surg* 1961; 42:497–506.
4. Duran CG, Gunning AJ: A method for placing a total homologous aortic valve in the subcoronary position. *Lancet* 1962; 2:488.
5. Ross DN: Homograft replacement of the aortic valve. *Lancet* 1962; 2:487.
6. Barratt-Boyes BG: Homograft aortic valve replacement in aortic incompetence and stenosis. *Thorax* 1964; 19:131–150.
7. Barratt-Boyes BG, Roche AHG, Whitlock RML: Six year review of the results of freehand aortic valve replacement using an antibiotic sterilized homograft valve. *Circulation* 1977; 55:353–361.
8. Khanna SK, Ross JK, Monro JL: Homograft aortic valve replacement: Seven years' experience with antibiotic- treated valves. *Thorax* 1981; 36:330–337.
9. Van Der Kamp AWM, Nauta J: Fibroblast function and the maintenance of the aortic valve matrix. *Cardiovasc Res* 1979; 13:167–172.
10. Somerville J, Saravalli O, Ross DN, et al: Long-term results of pulmonary autograft for aortic valve replacement. *Br Heart J* 1979; 42:533–540.
11. O'Brien M, Stafford EG, Gardner M, et al: The viable cryopreserved allograft aortic valve. *J Cardiac Surg* 1987; 1:153–167.
12. Angell WW, Shumway NE, Kosek JC: A 5-year study of viable aortic valve homografts. *J Thorac Cardiovasc Surg* 1972; 64:329–339.
13. Al-Janabi N, Gonzalez-Lavin L, Neirotti R, et al: Viability of fresh aortic valve homografts: A quantitative assessment. *Thorax* 1972; 27:83–86.
14. Gonzalez-Lavin L, O'Connell TX: Mitral valve replacement with viable aortic homograft valves. *Ann Thorac Surg* 1973; 15:592–600.
15. Al-Janabi N, Ross DN: Enhanced viability of fresh aortic homografts stored in nutrient medium. *Cardiovasc Res* 1973; 7:817–822.
16. Penta A, Qureshi S, Radley-Smith R, et al: Patient status 10 or more years after 'fresh' homograft replacement of the aortic valve. *Circulation* 1984; 70(suppl 1):182–186.
17. McGiffin DC, O'Brien MF, Stafford EG, et al: Long-term results of the viable cryopreserved allograft aortic valve: Continuing evidence for superior valve durability. *J Card Surg* 1988; 3:289–296.
18. O'Brien MF, Stafford EG, Gardner MAH, et al: The cryopreserved viable allograft aortic valves, in Yankah AC, Hetzer R, Yacoub MH, et al (eds): *Cardiac Valve Allografts 1962–1987.* Darmstadt, West Germany, Steinkopff Verlag, 1988, pp 311–321.
19. O'Brien MF, Johnston N, Stafford EG, et al: A study of the cells in the explanted viable cryopreserved allograft valve. *J Card Surg* 1988; 3:279–287.
20. Gavin JB, Barratt-Boyes BG, Hitchcock GC, et al: Histopathology of 'fresh' human aortic valve allografts. *Thorax* 1973; 28:482–487.
21. Armiger LC, Gavin JB, Barratt-Boyes BG: Histological assessment of orthotopic aortic valve leaflet allografts: Its role in selecting graft pre-treatment. *Pathology* 1983; 15:67–73.
22. Kosek JC, Iben AB, Shumway NE, et al: Morphology of fresh heart valve homografts. *Surgery* 1969; 66:269–274.
23. O'Brien MF, Stafford EG, Gardner MA, et al: A comparison of aortic valve replacement with viable cryopreserved and fresh allograft valves, with a note on chromosomal studies. *J Thorac Cardiovasc Surg* 1987; 94:812–823.
24. Ivert TSA, Dismukes WE, Cobbs CG, et al: Prosthetic valve endocarditis. *Circulation* 1984; 69:223–232.

25. Kirklin JK, Kirklin JW, Pacifico AD: Aortic valve endocarditis with aortic root abscess cavity: Surgical treatment with aortic valve homograft. *Ann Thorac Surg* 1988; 45:674–677.
26. Barratt-Boyes BG: Cardiothoracic surgery in the antipodes. *J Thorac Cardiovasc Surg* 1979; 78:804–822.
27. Thiede A, Timm C, Bernhard A, et al: Studies on the antigenicity of vital allogeneic valve leaflet transplants in immunogenetically controlled strain combinations. *Transplantation* 1978; 26:391–395.
28. Yankah AC, Feller AC, Thiede A, et al: Identification of surface antigens of endothelial cells of fresh preserved heart allografts: An indication for crossmatching for ABO and HLA antigen? (abstracted). *Thorac Cardiovasc Surg* 1986; 34:96.
29. Heslop BF, Wilson SE, Hardy BE: Antigenicity of aortic valve allografts. *Ann Surg* 1973; 177:301–306.
30. Yacoub M, Suitters A, Khaghani A, et al: Localization of major histocompatibility complex (HLA, ABC, and DR) antigens in aortic homografts, in Bodner E, Yacoub M (eds): *Biologic and Bioprosthetic Valves: Proceedings of the Third International Symposium.* New York, Yorke Medical Books, 1986, pp 65–72.
31. Mohri H, Reichenbach DD, Barnes RW, et al: Studies of antigenicity of the homologous aortic valve. *J Thorac Cardiovasc Surg* 1967; 54:564–572.
32. Yankah AC, Dreyer W, Wottge HU, et al: Kinetics of endothelial cells of preserved aortic valve allografts used for heterotopic transplantation in inbred rat strains, in Bodner E, Yacoub M (eds): *Biologic and Bioprosthetic Valves: Proceedings of the Third International Symposium.* New York, Yorke Medical Books, 1986, pp 73–87.
33. Balch CM, Karp RB: Blood group compatibility and aortic valve allotransplantation in man. *J Thorac Cardiovasc Surg* 1975; 70:256–259.
34. Yacoub M, in discussion, Yankah AC, Dreyer W, Wottge HU, et al: Kinetics of endothelial cells of preserved aortic valve allografts used for heterotopic transplantation in inbred rat strains, in Bodner E, Yacoub M (eds): *Biologic and Bioprosthetic Valves: Proceedings of the Third International Symposium.* New York, Yorke Medical Books, 1986, pp 73–87.
35. Al-Janabi N, Gibson K, Rose J, et al: Protein synthesis in fresh aortic and pulmonary valve allografts as an additional test for viability. *Cardiovasc Res* 1973; 7:247–250.
36. Yankah AC: Personal communication, September 1987.
37. Virdi IS, Munro JL, Ross JK: Aortic valve replacement with antibiotic- sterilized homograft valves: Eleven-year experience at Southampton, in Bodner E, Yacoub M (eds): *Biologic and Bioprosthetic Valves: Proceedings of the Third International Symposium.* New York, Yorke Medical Books, 1986, pp 29–37.
38. Clarke D: Personal communication, September 1986.
39. Bank H: Personal communication, September 1986.
40. Kirklin JK, Kirklin JW, Pacifico AD: Homograft replacement of the aortic valve. *Cardiol Clin* 1985; 3:329–341.
41. Somerville J, Ross DN: Homograft replacement of aortic root with reimplantation of coronary arteries. *Br Heart J* 1982; 47:473–482.
42. Donaldson RM, Ross DN: Homograft aortic root replacement for complicated prosthetic valve endocarditis. *Circulation* 1984; 70(suppl 1):178–181.
43. Lau JKH, Robles A, Cherian A, et al: Surgical treatment of prosthetic endocarditis. *J Thorac Cardiovasc Surg* 1984; 87:712–716.

44. McGiffin DC, O'Brien MF: A technique for aortic root replacement by an aortic allograft. *Ann Thorac Surg*, 1989; 47(4):625–627.
45. Dhalla N, Khaghani A, Radley-Smith R, et al: Early and long-term performance of aortic homograft root replacement, in Bodner E, Yacoub M (eds): *Biologic and Bioprosthetic Valves: Proceedings of the Third International Symposium*. New York, Yorke Medical Books, 1986, pp 7–13.
46. Clarke D: Transplantation techniques and the use of cryopreserved allograft cardiac valves. Presented at the Cryolife Inc Symposium Colorado, Beaver Creek, Sept 1986.
47. Heng MK, Barratt-Boyes BG, Agnew TM, et al: Isolated mitral replacement with stent-mounted antibiotic treated aortic allograft valves. *J Thorac Cardiovasc Surg* 1977; 74:230–237.
48. Yacoub MH, Kittle CF: A new technique for replacement of the mitral valve by a semilunar valve homograft. *J Thorac Cardiovasc Surg* 1969; 58:859–869.
49. Oh W, Somerville J, Ross DN, et al: Mitral valve replacement with preserved cadaveric aortic homografts. *J Thorac Cardiovasc Surg* 1973; 65:712–721.
50. Mankad PS, Khaghani A, Esposito G: Late results of mitral valve replacement using unstented antibiotic-sterilized aortic homografts, in Bodner E, Yacoub M (eds): *Biologic and Bioprosthetic Valves: Proceedings of the Third International Symposium*. New York, Yorke Medical Books, 1986, pp 47–57.
51. Robles A, Vaughan M, Lau JK, et al: Long-term assessment of aortic valve replacement with autologous pulmonary valve. *Ann Thorac Surg* 1985; 39:238–242.
52. Ross DN, Geens M: Heart valve replacement with pulmonary autografts, in Ionescu MJ, Ross DN, Wooler SH (eds): *Biological Tissue in Heart Valve Replacement*. Stoneham, Mass, Butterworths, 1972, pp 575–599.
53. Ross DN, Somerville J: Correction of pulmonary atresia with a homograft aortic valve. *Lancet* 1966; 2:1446–1447.
54. Marcelletti C, Mair DD: The Rastelli operation for transposition of the great arteries. *J Thorac Cardiovasc Surg* 1976; 72:427–434.
55. Bailey WW, Kirklin JW, Bargeron LM, et al: Late results with synthetic valved external conduits from venous ventricle to pulmonary arteries. *Circulation* 1977; 56(suppl 2):73–79.
56. Norwood WI, Freed MD, Rocchini AP, et al: Experience with valved conduits for repair of congenital cardiac lesions. *Ann Thorac Surg* 1977; 24:223–232.
57. Fontan F, Choussat A, Deville C, et al: Aortic valve homografts in the surgical treatment of complex cardiac malformations. *J Thorac Cardiovasc Surg* 1984; 87:649–657.
58. Di Carlo D, de Leval MR, Stark J: "Fresh," antibiotic sterilized aortic homografts in extra-cardiac valved conduits: Long-term results. *Thorac Cardiovasc Surg* 1984; 32:10–14.
59. Kay PH, Livi U, Robles A, et al: Pulmonary homograft, in Bodner E, Yacoub M (eds): *Biologic and Bioprosthetic Valves: Proceedings of the Third International Symposium*. New York, Yorke Medical Books, 1986, pp 58–64.

Surgical Treatment of Ventricular Arrhythmias

John M. Moran, M.D.

Professor of Surgery, University of Massachusetts Medical School, Worcester, Massachusetts

Several developments during the past decade have combined to create great interest in the operative treatment of ventricular tachyarrhythmias that are not controllable by drug therapy. Precise electrophysiologic diagnosis by means of endocardial catheter mapping has become available and, concomitantly, the ability to initiate and terminate tachycardias using extrastimulus techniques. The refinement of cardiopulmonary bypass and myocardial protection techniques have helped provide a milieu in which surgeons have been able to develop a variety of ablative techniques directed at the source(s) of arrhythmia; the extension of electrophysiologic studies to the operating room in the form of epicardial and endocardial mapping has provided new knowledge about arrhythmias and has helped guide their efforts. An appreciation of the characteristics and frequency of "sudden death," together with the success of cardiopulmonary resuscitation techniques, have provided a reservoir of patients in need of electrophysiologic diagnosis and either medical or surgical therapy, or their combination. Because of these various factors, the balance has shifted markedly in favor of a satisfactory result for patients who undergo surgery for the control of ventricular arrhythmia.

Background for Surgical Approach

Electrophysiologic Diagnosis

The basis for our current surgical approaches to ventricular tachyarrhythmia is the knowledge of cardiac electrophysiology, which has been afforded by the development and widespread use of invasive catheter techniques during the past decade; electrophysiology has become a fully established subspecialty within cardiology as a result. Some 70 years ago, Sir Thomas Lewis[1] first recorded from the canine epicardial surface the sequence of electrical activation in the ventricles. Fifteen years later, Barker and associates[2] were able to obtain and describe relatively complete epicardial activation sequences in the human heart. Durrer and associates,[3] 40 years after that, reported more details of epicardial, intramyocardial, and endocardial activation sequences and conduction velocities in a series of experiments on isolated human hearts. Based largely on their work, the normal sequence of electrical activation in the human heart has been delineated. An outgrowth of this has been the study of activation sequences in ventricular tachycardia (VT), which in turn has provided stimulus for surgical approaches to amelioration or cure of that condition.

Considerable debate has been generated concerning the precise electrical pathogenesis of ventricular arrhythmia, over whether foci of automaticity or the reentry phenomenon is the primary pathophysiologic etiology. Exhaustive study by many groups has provided evidence that the reentry phenomenon can be responsible for ventricular dysrhythmias. The main requirement for reentry is two adjacent pathways of conduction, with different characteristics of transmission, which are connected both proximally and distally in terms of the direction of myocardial excitation. Unidirectional block must exist such that an impulse can travel in only one direction along one pathway; there must be slow conduction such that the impulse traveling down the other, blocked pathway has time to recover excitability so that the impulse may reenter the circuit in a retrograde direction.[4] This mechanism has been demonstrated in isolated myocardial strips, in the intact dog heart, and more recently, in humans at the time of surgery.

Reentry pathways may be classified as "macro," being routed, for instance, through the atrioventricular conduction system, or "micro" in a syncytium of myocardium and scar at the edge of a ventricular aneurysm. The classic macro–reentry circuits associated with the Wolff-Parkinson-White syndrome are the best-understood and best-documented examples of this type of reentry and have been the most amenable to a surgically curative approach.

The induction of VT by programmed electrical stimulation (PES) has been considered as evidence that a reentry phenomenon exists. There is also evidence that some ventricular arrhythmias are generated from locally triggered activity, perhaps initiated by hypoxia, electrolyte abnormalities, or catecholamines. It is currently believed, however, that most VTs are due to reentry, and therefore that PES not only can reproduce such arrhythmias in predictable fashion but also can be utilized to terminate them.

The efforts made to establish this concept have logically led to sophisticated electrophysiologic catheter mapping, now routinely carried out in the electrophysiologic laboratory. The evolution of the laboratory demonstration of myocardial activation sequences and the initiation in humans of tachyarrhythmias by extrastimulus techniques has led to various forms of myocardial mapping in the exposed human heart at operation. Epicardial mapping was first performed in 1964 by Durrer et al.[5] to identify areas of chronic ischemia; Kaiser et al.[6] in 1970 performed epicardial mapping in patients with acute infarction to delineate areas of ischemia. Subsequently, Kastor et al.[7] in 1972 studied the sites of origin of ventricular ectopic beats using epicardial mapping in arrhythmias produced either by digitalis or by electrical stimulus. These studies laid the background for epicardial mapping in clinical ventricular arrhythmia first reported by Fontaine et al.[8] in 1974. In the course of the subsequent decade, epicardial, transmural, and endocardial mapping have taken hold as an important aid in the surgery of ventricular arrhythmia.

The ability to induce and to terminate a ventricular arrhythmia using PES has become an invaluable tool for evaluating the effects of various interventions on the dysrhythmia, especially pharmacologic and surgical therapy. The concept that a drug that can prevent induction of a tachycardia that had been readily inducible in a drug-free state, could be a satisfactory marker for long-term management under the appropriate drug therapy, was first documented by Wu et al.[9] of Rosen's laboratory. They described a series of patients in whom appropriate drug therapy rendered VT noninducible or quickly self-terminating. This effective approach was rapidly confirmed by other workers[10]; such extrastimulus testing has become a bedrock in the clinical management of ventricular arrhythmias. There are, however, exceptions in the case of certain drugs, such as amiodarone, whereby certain patients may have inducible VT and yet have a good clinical response to the drug. In a collective review, Horowitz et al.[11] compiled the experience from six centers employing PES techniques to select drug therapy for recurrent sustained VT; 84% of patients for whom a drug could render the VT noninducible remained free of recurrent VT for over 1 year. If such a drug could not be found, patients fared poorly, with more than 75% having recurrences of arrhythmia, and with a mortality more than twice as great as in the successfully treated group. Ventricular tachycardia can be initiated in nearly all patients using electrical stimuli. Not all, however, may have VT initiated with ease by right ventricular free wall or apical pacing, and may require stimulation of the septum or the outflow tract or near some other site of origin of the VT. Left ventricular pacing may be required and is performed routinely in some centers.[11]

Endocardial Catheter Mapping

The activation sequence as well as the origin of VT can be evaluated by means of multiple catheters inserted under fluoroscopic guidance in the electrophysiologic laboratory. An area from which the earliest depolarization can be recorded appears to be an important marker for the site of origin of the arrhythmia. Historically, this technique has been used to delineate bypass tracts in patients with the Wolff-Parkinson-White syndrome, as well as to characterize sinus node function and locate ectopic atrial pacemakers. When located, the earliest ventricular endocardial activation site should slightly precede the beginning of the surface QRS complex from several leads. Up to a dozen sites within the left ventricle and half a dozen within the right ventricle can be thus mapped and an activation sequence derived. Practices vary from institution to institution, some relying heavily on these preoperative findings to guide an endocardial resection, whereas other groups do not utilize it. Electrophysiologic study following surgery is performed before hospital discharge; if an inducible arrhythmia persists, repeated studies are performed when various drug serum levels are therapeutic until satisfactory drug control of the arrhythmia is achieved. With current surgical techniques, however, VTs of a high percentage of patients are rendered noninducible and they are discharged without drug treatment.

Patient Population

Although the great majority of patients undergoing electrophysiologic surgery for ventricular arrhythmia have ischemic heart disease as the basic etiology, others are seen occasionally who have important, albeit unusual or even rare, causes of arrhythmia requiring surgery.

Nonischemic Heart Disease

One of the most interesting of the unusual cardiac conditions giving rise to VT is right ventricular dysplasia. In its most complete form the "parchment right ventricle" is known as Uhl's syndrome, in which epicardium and endocardium come into contact without any intervening myocardium.[12] There are lesser degrees of this syndrome, which has been best studied by Guiraudon et al.,[13] who have classified it as "arrhythmogenic right ventricular dysplasia." The surgery for this entity requires detailed intraoperative mapping, localization of the source of the arrhythmia, and excision of the area involved, insofar as anatomically possible. Guiraudon et al.[13] have perhaps the largest experience with a variety of other clinical conditions causing VT. These take the form of nonobstructive cardiomyopathies and idiopathic ventricular aneurysms, and some patients have spontaneous tachycardias that can only be described as idiopathic since they are unassociated with aneurysm or other detectable abnormality. If such foci are located in the septum, the result of operation is not likely to be successful.

Granulomatous disease of the heart, most notably sarcoidosis, can result in recurrent VT and "sudden death." We have had experience with two such cases. In one VT was localized to the papillary muscles, with a successful surgical result. The other had multiple morphology tachycardia due to diffuse myocardial sarcoidosis; medical and surgical therapy ultimately failed.[14] Others have had a similar experience.

A not uncommon etiology of VT is previous surgery for congenital heart disease that required incision in the right ventricular outflow tract. Many of these cases can be handled with drugs, but occasionally surgery and excision of right ventricular scar may become necessary.

Another type of ventricular arrhythmia with some surgical implications is the long QT interval, described in 1957 by Jervell and Lang-Neilson.[15] This was originally described as a component of a clinical entity that also included congenital deafness and syncopal attacks due to ventricular fibrillation (VF) associated with physical or emotional stress. Subsequently, the long QT syndrome was described in patients following acute myocardial infarction who subsequently experienced a high incidence of sudden death due to VF, as in children with the congenital form of the long QT syndrome. It has been suggested by James et al.[16] that the etiology is a neuritis of the cardiac conduction system, perhaps due to a viral infectious process. The ventricular arrhythmia most often associated with the long QT syndrome is a chaotic type of rapid VT with a changing electrical axis that appears on rhythm strips as an undulating pattern, lacking the uniformity usually seen with records of VT. This has been named *torsade des pointes.* A not infrequent cause of torsade is use of medications that prolong ventricular repolarization, such as quinidine. This has led to the observation that this condition probably represents an abnormality in myocardial repolarization, as contrasted with other types of VT, which are thought to be abnormalities of depolarization.[17] This has fostered interest in efforts to modify cardiac innervation; studies in animals have shown that right stellate ganglion resection or left stellate ganglion stimulation results in a prolonged QT interval and increased T-wave amplitude. Consequently, left stellate ganglion resection has been utilized with success in small numbers of patients with the long QT syndrome.[18] Another mode of treatment for the long QT interval syndrome has been the automatic internal difibrillator, which has met with perhaps more success than stellate ganglionectomy.

Ischemic Heart Disease

The remainder of this chapter will be devoted to the larger and more homogeneous category of patients who have ischemic heart disease as the etiology for ventricular arrhythmia.

Patient Population at Risk.—Although significant gains have been made in the public health sphere in recent years, directed toward the prevention of coronary heart disease, it is still the leading cause of death in the United States; over a million patients per year die of diseases of the cardiovascular system. About two thirds of these patients die of cardiac involvement, and it is estimated that approximately 400,000 patients per year die suddenly. The true incidence may never be known, but the evidence suggests that most sudden deaths are arrhythmic in nature. One of the early studies, that of Schaffer and Cobb in 1975,[19] the Seattle experience, revealed that approximately 75% of patients experiencing sudden death had documented VF. The great success of cardiopulmonary resuscitation is a matter of record; it has helped to create a reservoir of patients who, according to the tenor of our times, become candidates for electrophysiologic investigation, drug therapy, and/or surgical intervention.

Patient Selection for Surgery.—The typical patient coming to surgery for refractory ventricular arrhythmia has had several episodes of wide QRS tachycardia causing multiple hospital admissions for diagnosis and treatment. Infarction responsible for setting this chain of events into motion may have occurred months or even years before the arrhythmic event, in our experience as much as 30 years prior. The patient is then subjected to electrophysiologic study using PES. If a drug can be found that makes VT no longer inducible, he will be discharged on this drug regimen and followed up closely. If such a drug cannot be found or if there are compelling reasons for surgery, an antiarrhythmia operation will be recommended; this is usually combined with myocardial revascularization. The most common such compelling surgical indication is severe three-vessel disease and/

TABLE 1.
Evaluating the Patient With Recurrent Sustained VT and Survivors of Out-of-Hospital VF*

All Patients	
Step 1	Documentation of tachycardia QRS morphology in 12 surface ECG leads
	Analysis of QRS morphologies from all documented tachycardia episodes searching for multiple morphologies
	Careful drug history emphasizing side effects and serum drug levels
Step 2	Admission to coronary care unit for withdrawal of antiarrhythmic drug therapy
	Complete electrophysiologic study under control conditions

Patients With No Inducible VT

Step 3	Study multiple sites
	Right ventricular outflow
	Left ventricle
	Repeat study after isoproterenol infusion
	Conduct exercise test for VT provocation
Step 4	Discharge without long-term antiarrhythmic therapy

Patients With Inducible VT

Step 3	Serial drug studies at maximum tolerated dose under steady-state conditions
	Conventional drugs
	Experimental drugs
	Determination of serum level of drug resulting in efficacious response

Drug Responders

Step 4	Exercise testing to document control
	Discharge with long-term oral therapy
	Frequent outpatient follow-up with serum drug level determinations to adjust dosages

Nonresponders

Step 4	Diagnostic cardiac catheterization to assess operability
Step 5	Endocardial resection (patients with reasonable surgical risk)
	Long-term amiodarone therapy (high-risk surgical patients)
Step 6	In patients receiving amiodarone with spontaneously recurring VT
	Implantable cardioversion device
	Automatic antitachycardia burst pacemaker
	Reassessment of operability

*Adapted from Kehoe RF, Loeb JM, Zheutlin T, et al: Invasive electrophysiologic studies in directing therapy for malignant ventricular arrhythmia, in Roberts AJ (ed): *Coronary Artery Surgery: Application of New Technologies*. Chicago, Year Book Medical Publishers, 1983, p 243.

or tight left main coronary stenosis. Occasionally, other complications of previous infarction, such as severe mitral regurgitation or a hemodynamically significant ventricular aneurysm, may also provide a contraindication for the full course of selection for surgery by means of drug trial and PES.

Another distinct type of patient is one who has survived out-of-hospital VF. In this group, subsequent PES will usually result in degeneration of VT rather quickly into VF, requiring countershock. An interesting subgroup of patients with VT are those in whom a clinically benign and self-limited arrhythmia may be converted by drug therapy to one with serious ramifications.[20, 21] This situation is unmasked by a control, or drug-free, study after a period of continuous monitoring in the coronary care unit so that antiarrhythmic drugs can safely be withdrawn. It must be emphasized that complete electrophysiologic study is necessary to fully characterize the sinoatrioventricular conduction system and not merely to focus on inducibility of VT. It is not the purpose in this chapter to describe all of the many nuances of electrophysiologic study but rather to focus on the many facets of surgery. Practices vary somewhat from institution to institution, but the algorithm in Table 1 sets forth one approach to selection of patients for operation.

A significant subgroup of patients are those with sudden death and documented out-of-hospital VF who are found on cardiac catheterization to have severe coronary stenosis, often of the left main coronary artery or the proximal left anterior descending artery. Characteristically, they have no wall motion abnormality, as do others having experienced "sudden death"; this correlates with a history free of myocardial infarction. Usually, PES is not effective in inducing VT. On the other hand, exercise testing may result in VF caused by ischemia, thus duplicating the situation requiring out-of-hospital resuscitation.[14]

Surgery for Ventricular Arrhythmias

Evolution of Surgical Approaches

In an earlier surgical era, recurrent supraventricular tachycardias were treated with bilateral thoracic sympathectomy with some success.[22, 23] The use of thoracic sympathectomy for recurrent VT is based on a theory that myocardial catecholamines may be responsible for initiation of ventricular ectopia. Animal studies reveal that division of the cardiac sympathetic nerve supply will diminish the incidence of VF after coronary artery ligation.[24] In a number of case reports, sympathectomy was found to be effective in diminishing the incidence of recurrent VT.[25–27]

The first direct surgical attack on the heart expressly for the control of intractable VT was taken by Bailey in 1956 and reported by Couch[28] in 1959. In 1956, Likoff and Bailey[29] reported ventricular aneurysmectomy in seven patients, five of whom had recurrent ventricular arrhythmias; three were relieved by surgery. That feat is even more remarkable when one considers that those early operations were done without the benefit of cardiopulmonary bypass. Previous to that, the association between ventricular aneurysm and arrhythmia had surfaced only rarely in the literature, having first been described by Parkinson et al.[30] in 1938. In one of the first large series of operations for ventricular aneurysm in the modern era of cardiac surgery, Loop et al.[31] reported VT as a major presenting problem in 7% of patients with aneurysm and as a sole indication for operation in 3%. In our early experience, 10% of patients undergoing surgery for aneurysm presented with VT as a primary indication.[32]

Beginning in 1969, ventricular aneurysmectomy as the sole surgical treatment for intractable arrhythmia was described from a number of sources.[33-39] The results of operation were highly variable, with mortality ranging from 0% to 50% and with variable numbers of patients requiring continued drug therapy. Subsequently, myocardial revascularization alone was applied in an aura of optimism that the arrhythmogenic foci would somehow be rendered neutral, but not long after the initial reports it became apparent that this was not curative and that most survivors required long-term antiarrhythmia drug therapy.[40-43]

In the first few years of the coronary surgery era, it was widely believed that the combination of revascularization and aneurysmectomy, and in certain instances the use of the intra-aortic balloon pump, would provide a surgical solution to the problem of recurrent and refractory VT, but this approach was also found wanting.[32, 44-46] For example, in our early experience with this combination therapy in 15 patients in whom arrhythmia was the primary surgical indication, the postoperative hospital mortality was 33%, and the late mortality was 27%, all deaths being in the sudden death category.[47] Therefore, it was apparent that the problem was far from being solved; rather, these failures served to focus further attention on a difficult problem. The evolution of electrophysiologic methods described above and the early surface mapping attempts in dogs and in humans[6, 7] suggested the use of epicardial mapping for intractable ventricular arrhythmia. This was first performed by Fontaine et al.,[8] who used the findings of epicardial mapping to guide incisions, or limited excisions in an attempt to ablate the source of arrhythmia. Spurrell et al.[48, 49] used operative mapping to guide bundle-branch division and, subsequently, epicardial incision designed to interrupt reentry pathways. Wittig and Boineau[50] in 1975 reported in three patients the successful use of epicardial as well as transmural and endocardial mapping by means of plunge electrodes, as a guide for epicardially directed incision and excision. Subsequently, we reported a similar series of five patients with results much improved over aneurysmectomy and bypass alone, but less than ideal because of the continued need for antiarrhythmic therapy.[47] During this period, Guiraudon and associates[51] were developing the operation of encircling endocardial ventriculotomy (EEV), which was a deep incision from endocardium to just short of epicardium, beyond the border zone of aneurysmal scar, designed to isolate the arrhythmogenic area; this did not necessarily require guidance by mapping. An important conceptual and technical advance was provided by

Harken and associates,[52] who performed detailed preoperative endocardial mapping, followed by extensive operative endocardial mapping of the open beating ventricle during sustained VT; they used these findings to direct an excision of a limited target area of endocardial scar. Subsequently, utilizing a similar operative mapping approach, we elected to remove all visible postinfarction endocardial scar, taking into full consideration the early points of activation delineated by mapping.[53] There were several reasons for this approach to a combined map-directed and visually directed endocardial resection. Early in our experience we had demonstrated that tachycardias of differing morphologies can arise from geographically separate areas of endocardium; many patients have multiple clinical morphologies of VT recorded preoperatively, all of which may not be inducible at the time of operation. It is known that life-threatening arrhythmias may occur many years after infarction, even as late as 30 years in our experience. Therefore, we believe that dense scar left behind is a matrix for future threat of sudden death and should be removed, provided it can be done without additional risk to the patient.

Another form of ablative therapy, the cryolesion, has been used either solely or in conjunction with other methods to eradicate arrhythmogenic foci or pathways.[54–56] These cryolesions are created with metallic probes that transmit cold generated by either liquid nitrogen or expanding nitrous oxide. This has been shown to produce limited infarction with a very homogeneous type of healing, unlike the random and heterogeneous scar produced by ischemic infarction. Such cryolesions are usually employed in strategic locations, such as papillary muscle or scar abutting the mitral or aortic anulus. Further, Guiraudon et al.[57] have described the encircling use of the cryolesion, which is intended to accomplish in a somewhat safer way the isolation of arrhythmogenicity for which EEV had previously been designed.

More recently still, the neodymium–yttrium aluminum garnet (Nd-YAG) laser has been used to ablate endocardial scar in the normothermic open beating heart during induced ventricular tachycardia.[58, 59] The heart returns to sinus rhythm when the responsible area is located and ablated; aortic cross clamping has not been necessary. This is an exciting new method and may well become the method of choice for ablating arrhythmogenic foci or pathways.

Intraoperative Management

In the usual, reasonably stable patient being prepared for electrophysiologic surgery, antiarrhythmic drug therapy is discontinued on the evening before operation. Conventional premedication is utilized, and on arrival in the operating room, ECG leads I, aV_F, V_{4R}, and V_5 are established, along with two large intravenous lines, a radial artery monitoring line, and a multipurpose pulmonary artery catheter. Interestingly, in this experience with patients with arrhythmia, our concerns about induction of arrhythmia by passage of the Swan-Ganz catheter through the right ventricle have proved groundless: no significant arrhythmias have been seen in the entire experience due to this cause. The ECG leads are connected to a multichannel oscilloscope and rapid-writing recorder with the capability for storage on tape. Anesthesia is induced with diazepam (Valium) or thiopental and maintained with fentanyl, halothane, isoflurane (Forane), or enflurane, and the use of antiarrhythmic drugs is avoided. After sternotomy, the patient is then heparinized and cannulated but not placed on bypass until hypotension incident to arrhythmia induction occurs. Normothermia or slight hyperthermia is maintained to facilitate arrhythmia induction.

To standardize epicardial recording data, the entire surface of both ventricles is arbitrarily divided into a grid comprising 64 individual sites (Fig 1). An intramural bipolar reference electrode comprising two stainless steel pins 1 mm apart is placed on the anterior surface of the right ventricle. A complete epicardial map in sinus rhythm is then obtained, coordinating surface anatomy with the epicardial diagram, in search of areas of poor depolarization patterns indicating slow conduction.

Programmed electrical stimulation is then initiated by means of an epicardial pacing wire. Single and double premature stimuli and burst pacing modes are used, all at approximately twice the diastolic stimulation threshold. On occasion, when induction of VT proves difficult, isoproterenol is given to increase ventricular irritability. A moderate degree of ventricular distention also appears to facilitate inducibility. If VT is too rapid for accurate mapping or if it degenerates into VF, procainamide is useful in slowing

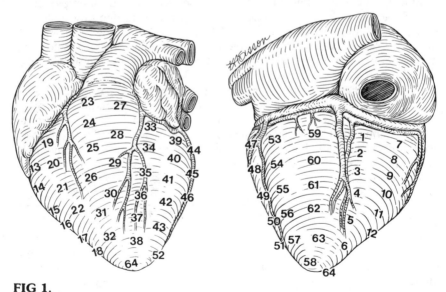

FIG 1.
Sixty-four arbitrary epicardial points are selected for surface mapping, beginning posteriorly to the left of the septum at the atrioventricular junction and ending at the left ventricular apex. (From Moran JM: Surgical management of malignant ventricular arrhythmia. *Crit Care Q* 1984; 7:53. Used by permission.)

the rhythm and stabilizing it. Careful attention is paid to the tachycardia morphology to determine if the arrhythmia induced is similar to that recorded during spontaneous VT and/or that induced during PES preoperatively. Complete epicardial mapping during VT can then be carried out in 2 or 3 minutes using a bipolar fingertip electrode.

Special attention is paid to areas of slowed and slurred conduction, but especially to areas of earliest depolarization in reference to the surface QRS. Attention is also given to the recordings from aneurysmal borders and from both sides of the interventricular septum anteriorly and posteriorly, as they are the most common exit points. If more than one tachycardia had been present clinically or produced by preoperative PES, attempts are made to reproduce each morphology. For each one, the earliest recorded site of epicardial activity is noted.

The ventricle is then opened through the center of the aneurysm, making the incision no longer than absolutely necessary for accurate endocardial mapping. This precaution is taken because occasionally VT has become noninducible after ventriculotomy owing to interruption of a reentry pathway at the border of the aneurysm.

In our initial experience, the fingertip electrode was used in concentric circles using clock coordinates in reference to the incision, 12 o'clock being cephalad for anterior ventriculotomies and toward the cardiac apex with inferior wall ventriculotomies. Thus, 12 circumferential points were mapped at alphabetized increments 1-cm in depth from the edge of the ventriculotomy. This method had the drawback of being somewhat time-consuming; the induced VT would often cease or change in character and polarity. A partial solution to this problem was the development of a multiple-pole probe, which simultaneously provides bipolar electrograms at six points, thus materially speeding the endocardial map, which can now be obtained in 3 to 5 minutes if VT is sustained[60] (Figs 2 and 3).

In approximately 20% of our cases, the clinical or preoperative PES arrhythmia is not inducible at surgery, owing in part to the antiarrhythmia effects of general anesthesia. In this instance, pace mapping is utilized: a bipolar pencil electrode stimulates the myocardium in various locations in search of a morphology that most closely resembles that of the clinical arrhythmia. Not infrequently, completely different morphologies of VT can be identified from the same sites on the endocardial map (Figs 3 and 4). Careful note is made of these, and the excision of endocardial scar in these areas is carried somewhat more deeply than in other areas. It is common to have two or more distinctly separate areas of dense endocardial scar within the ventricle, each one associated with previous infarction; it is not uncommon to demonstrate a different morphology of VT arising from each area. The typical patient with anteroseptal aneurysm has a large flat sheet of dense white scar extending over half to two thirds of the septum.

From the beginning of our experience, we have been convinced that the most logical approach to endocardial ablation for arrhythmia is to remove all postinfarction scar, especially at border zones, insofar as is possible. The time required for removal of all or most of the scar is insignificantly longer

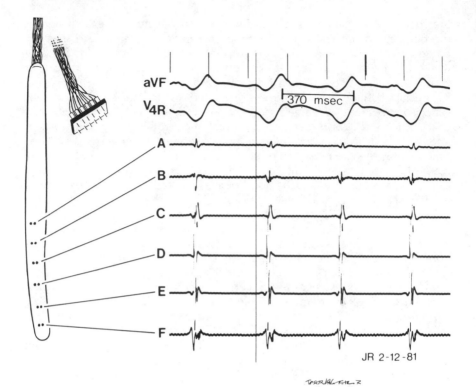

aVF

V₄R

370 msec

A

B

C

D

E

F

JR 2-12-81

FIG 2.
Multiple-pole probe. Each electrode is separated by 1 mm, the pairs by 1 cm. This is an example of recordings taken simultaneously from normal-appearing myocardium. Note that depolarization is nearly simultaneous, and that the signals are well delineated. (From Loeb JM, Kehoe RF, Moran JM: Intraoperative electrophysiologic approach to the patient with recurrent life threatening ventricular tachyarrhythmia, in Roberts AJ (ed): *Coronary Artery Surgery: Application of New Technologies*. Chicago, Year Book Medical Publishers, 1983, p 221. Used by permission.)

than that required for a limited endocardial resection. Our practice has been to proceed immediately after mapping with the endocardial resection, removing all visible and accessible endocardial scar, with special attention to any area(s) of earliest depolarization during one or more of the induced tachycardia patterns. If the clinical VT has a left bundle branch block morphology, and operative mapping suggests a right ventricular source, the surgeons should be prepared to explore the right ventricle and excise endocardium as appropriate (Figs 5 and 6).

For improved operating conditions, systemic hypothermia is instituted, the aorta is cross clamped, and cold cardioplegia solution is injected into the root of the aorta. Some authors have advocated keeping the heart normothermic, either in fibrillation or the beating state, performing the en-

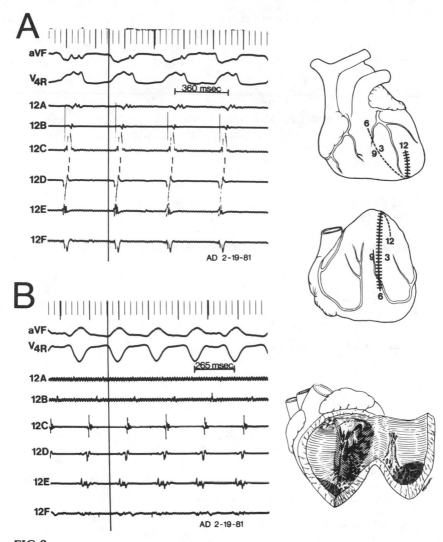

FIG 3.
Note different activation sequence in case 1 **(A)** and case 2 **(B).** Slurred tracings at points 12A and 12B in case 2, at border zone of apical aneurysm anteriorly, suggest that this is an early point of activation. (From Loeb JM, Kehoe RF, Moran JM: Intraoperative electrophysiologic approach to the patient with recurrent life threatening ventricular tachyarrhythmia, in Roberts AJ (ed): *Coronary Artery Surgery: Application of New Technologies.* Chicago, Year Book Medical Publishers, 1983, p 221. Used by permission.)

docardial resection and then checking the results by attempting to reinduce VT. Our feeling is that such findings, either pro or con, may not stand the test of time; many patients with ultimately successful surgery proved by noninducibility at postoperative PES, and by the test of time, have had recurrent VT in the immediate postoperative period. Therefore, it would seem that such added effort under conditions of cardiopulmonary bypass may not bear fruit.

Some authors prefer to perform coronary revascularization, when appropriate, immediately after mapping is completed to provide better myocardial preservation through the various grafts as they are applied. In all

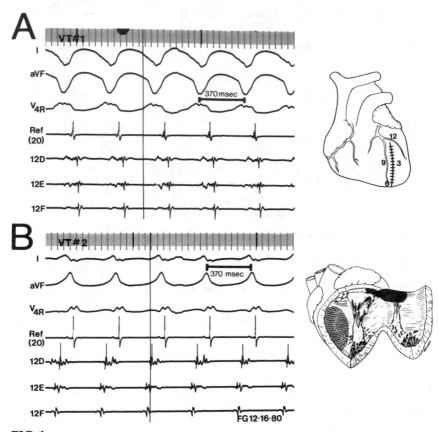

FIG 4.
Three of six bipolar leads in use. Note early activation of ventricular tachycardia (VT) in case 2 **(B)** in areas 12E and 12F, high on septum anteriorly, whereas in case 1 **(A),** activation in the same area is delayed, with completely different configuration. (From Loeb JM, Kehoe RF, Moran JM: Intraoperative electrophysiologic approach to the patient with recurrent life threatening ventricular tachyarrhythmia, in Roberts AJ (ed): *Coronary Artery Surgery: Application of New Technologies.* Chicago, Year Book Medical Publishers, 1983, p 221. Used by permission.)

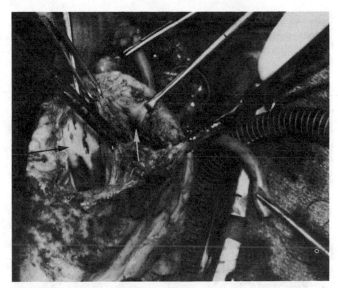

FIG 5.
Open right and left ventricles, taken from head of operating table. This patient had a left bundle-branch-block pattern of ventricular tachycardia, with earliest activation over right side of septum near the apex. *White arrow* indicates scar to be excised from the right ventricular apex; *black arrow* indicates a typical sheet of postinfarction endocardial scar in the left ventricle.

probability the exact sequence is of little importance. Our practice is to perform grafting after endocardial resection and aneurysm closure; 90% of our patients have been so grafted, with an average of 2.8 grafts per patient, ranging from one to five grafts. Approximately 10% of our patients have required mitral valve replacement.[61] This occurs in the setting of postinfarction mitral regurgitation of severe degree and also when the earliest point of activation is the base or the body of severely scarred papillary muscle.

This approach seems radical to some, and lesser measures have been described, such as an endocardial incision around the base of the posteromedial papillary muscle, either end being close to the mitral valve anulus and being supplemented by a cryolesion at each end of the incision.[62] We have found that postoperative inducibility of VT is associated primarily with inferior wall infarction and papillary muscle that has been left behind in favor of lesser procedures than complete excision and valve replacement.

Recently, Landymore[63] has described reconstruction of the papillary muscle after transection at the base, using transmural suture techniques. Following completion of the definitive part of the operation, right atrial and ventricular pacing wires are placed. They are useful not only for postoperative pacing, for the diagnosis of atrial and ventricular dysrhythmias, and

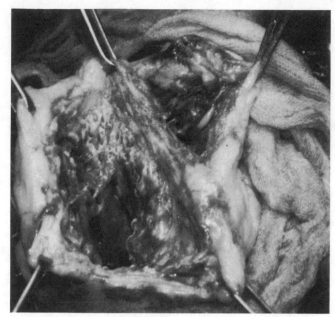

FIG 6.
View after completion of extended endocardial resection in both right and left ventricles.

for cardioversion by way of rapid pacing, but also for use during predischarge PES study.

Current Surgical Approaches and Results

The earliest procedures developed as a direct surgical attack on sources of ventricular arrhythmia are no longer used, except perhaps under special circumstances. These include the epicardially based incisions or excisions of areas found to be epicardial breakthrough points in VT,[47–50] and the EEV originally described by Guiraudon et al.[51] The results of epicardial incisions and excisions, although superior to those of revascularization and aneurysmectomy alone, proved to be unsatisfactory in comparison with subsequently developed procedures. The EEV is no longer used in the form originally described; Ungerleider and Cox and associates,[64–67] in a series of laboratory and clinical studies, have documented not only the positive effect of electrical isolation by this procedure but also the deleterious effects on ventricular function and hemodynamics. The operation may still be useful, however, in modified, limited form such as that described by Cox[62] for isolation of an arrhythmogenic area of the inferior wall, to include the papillary muscle. The procedures currently in favor are map-directed limited endocardial resection; extended endocardial resection (EER), with or without map guidance; the creation of cryolesions, either in special target areas or in an encircling mode; and the recently introduced

Nd-YAG laser, which has emerged as an interesting method of endocardial scar ablation.

Map-Directed Limited Endocardial Resection

The method first described by Harken et al.[52] depends heavily on preoperative as well as intraoperative endocardial mapping. In instances where arrhythmia is either not inducible or mappable at operation, those authors felt comfortable in excising an area 2 to 4 cm in diameter from an area located as a site of origin by endocardial mapping studies. In a subsequent report of 107 patients who had undergone a limited resection of this type, they reported a 30-day mortality of 9% and a 28% incidence of inducibility before discharge.[68] There were two late sudden deaths, most likely a result of recurrent arrhythmia. The VTs of seven patients remained inducible despite medication, but five had no clinical recurrence. The overall success rate was considered to be 85%, a figure that includes all cases rendered noninducible by drug therapy. The degree of success of this type of limited endocardial resection was confirmed by other workers: operative mortality is approximately 8% to 12%, postoperative inducibility of VT ranges from 22% to 45%, and 85% to 90% of patients are arrhythmia free over the short term, with or without antiarrhythmia medications.[69–72]

EER

In our initial report of a homogeneous experience of attempted removal of all postinfarction endocardial scar in 40 patients, the operative mortality was 10%, primarily caused by low cardiac output and/or hemorrhage incident to reoperation.[53] Among the 36 survivors at 3 to 36 months' follow-up, 91% of patients who underwent postoperative PES had noninducible VTs, 92% of survivors were free of arrhythmia without drug therapy, and the remaining three patients, VTs were well controlled by antiarrhythmic drugs. With further follow-up and an expanded series of 79 patients, now including more in high-risk subgroups (eg, inferior wall infarction), the operative mortality was 12% and the postoperative inducibility rate among 61 patients was 20%; all but two patients with inducible VT were now successfully treated with medication.[73]

Thus, as a result of EER, 96% of patients having postoperative PES could be rendered free of induced arrhythmia; overall, 17% of patients required subsequent drug treatment. In late follow-up, 59 (86%) of 69 survivors were arrhythmia free at 27 ± 15 months. Among the 10 patients having an arrhythmic event, nine (90%) had had inducible VTs, vs. two patients (4%) among 49 whose VTs had not been. Thus, once again the highly specific nature of postoperative inducibility as a marker for subsequent arrhythmia events has been demonstrated. Figures 7 and 8, respectively, show the actuarial survival and arrhythmia free survival at 5 years.

To assess the effect of EER on ventricular performance, we analyzed data from preoperative and postoperative nuclear ventriculograms in 43 patients.[74] In patients with aneurysms, as well as in those with akinetic wall motion abnormality alone, the extent of endocardial resection did not sig-

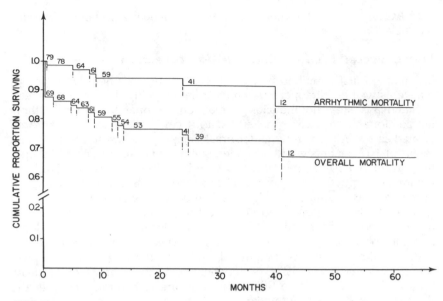

FIG 7.
Actuarial overall mortality, and that caused by arrhythmia, in 79 patients undergoing extended endocardial resection, to 65 months. Overall survival was 68%, with 15% from arrhythmia.

nificantly affect the ejection fraction; slight to moderate improvement was documented in both patients with aneurysm and patients without aneurysm.

Other groups of investigators performing complete resection of endocardial scar, with or without mapping, have also demonstrated improved results. Lawrie et al.,[75] after an initial experience with limited map-directed endocardial resection, in which the failure rate was 33%, reported their experience with extended resection: no recurrent arrhythmias were seen in 23 consecutive patients, and only one of 37 surviving patients had inducible VT. They also advocate the liberal use of cryolesions, including those applied to both sides of the septum, in cases with documented septal and right ventricular arrhythmic pathways. Landymore and associates[76] have described the results of complete visually directed endocardial resection in a series of ten patients. There was no operative mortality, and two late deaths were unrelated to arrhythmia. All patients were alive at mean follow-up of 17 months, without clinical arrhythmia; one patient had had inducible VT postoperatively and was successfully treated with medication.

Thus, it appears from these various reports, in aggregate, that an EER with or without mapping provides improved results over a limited, map-directed endocardial resection, without added morbidity or mortality. Presumably, this is so because remaining endocardial scar has the potential for generating future arrhythmia.

The issue of prophylactic endocardial resection arises during surgery for ventricular aneurysm in patients who have not experienced arrhythmia as a major clinical problem. Since endocardial scar left behind may subsequently become a source of arrhythmia and since reoperation for arrhythmia in patients having previously undergone aneurysm resection is a highly significant risk factor,[53] we have elected to take the approach of performing endocardial resection in this setting, provided there is no added risk to the patient. Thirteen patients have been so treated, without added morbidity, with full realization that the true value of such prophylactic resection is unknown. The decision to do this rests with the individual surgeon and will depend on the anatomic features in any given case.

Many patients, especially those with a history of inferior wall infarction, have involvement of the papillary muscles, usually the posteromedial papillary muscle. If significant mitral regurgitation is present, the decision to combine the antiarrhythmia operation with mitral valve replacement is straightforward. The decision becomes much more difficult when mitral competence exists, and the base or body of the papillary muscle is shown to be a site of early activation in one or more morphologies of VT. In our experience, the highest incidence of failure to eradicate the arrhythmia has been in those patients in whom endocardial scar has been left behind, in association with a papillary muscle. Lesser measures such as partial incisions of the base of the papillary muscle, and cross-hatching incisions of

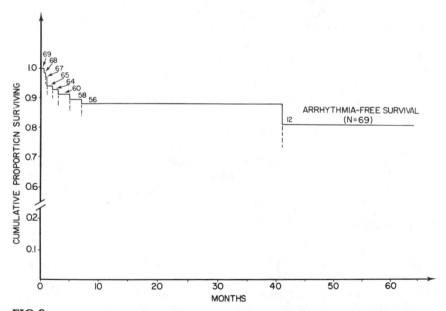

FIG 8.
Freedom from arrhythmia in 69 survivors of extended endocardial resection. Note the significant rate of freedom from late arrhythmia recurrence. Arrhythmia-free survival at 65 months is 82%.

the muscle body, have not been effective in arrhythmia control. Therefore, our approach has been to consider mitral valve replacement (MVR) in such patients.[60] Among nine such operations in which MVR was added to EER, there has been one operative mortality; all the remaining patients have remained free of inducible VT and arrhythmia. Among less radical approaches to this problem are the application of cryolesions to the base and body of the papillary muscle(s) and the combination of an encircling incision and cryolesion suggested by Cox.[62] The logical approach of complete transection of papillary muscle at its base, with reimplantation, as advocated by Landymore et al.,[63, 76] has been successful in arrhythmia ablation in 15 cases. Whether this method and that of Cox will prove superior to papillary muscle resection and valve replacement awaits further evaluation. These concepts are attractive not only because valve replacement may be avoided but also because the subvalvular mechanism remains intact and can exert its beneficial influence on ventricular performance in these patients, nearly all of whom have impaired function.

Cryolesions

The application of a freezing probe to myocardium causes a reversible injury at higher temperatures, e.g., −5°C to −10°C, which may be helpful in localizing a potential arrhythmogenic focus, which may then be ablated by lowering the temperature to −60°C for 2 minutes. Such cryolesions create a sharply defined area of homogeneous scar that is not in itself arrhythmogenic but is relatively inert and capable of interrupting conduction, whether it be orthodromic or aberrant. Harrison et al.[77] reported its use to ablate the His bundle; Gallagher et al.[78] first reported its use in VT. Cox[79] has utilized cryolesions liberally in "dangerous areas," e.g., about mitral and aortic anulus and papillary muscles.[79] A number of investigators have liberally combined the cryolesion with other methods of ablation, claiming added advantage. Perhaps the primary advantage is the ability to interrupt reentrant pathways in such sensitive areas as papillary muscle and those proximate to the mitral or aortic anuli or the conduction system. An innovative use of the cryolesion is the "encircling cryoablation" of Guiraudon et al.,[57] in which a series of lesions are created at the border zone of infarction to isolate it and render reentrant pathways nonconductive. Wyndham et al.[80] have successfully ablated septal sites of origin of VT by applying cryolesions to both right and left ventricular sides of the septum.

Laser Ablation

The continuous-wave Nd-YAG laser has characteristics that allow precise control of tissue penetration that can be adjusted by manipulating power and time exposure of the laser beam. There is substantial forward scatter of energy, unlike that associated with the CO_2 and argon laser beams. The use of this technique was first described by Mesnildry et al.[58]

In a series of five patients, and ten more reported in an addendum, Selle et al.[59] utilized the Nd-YAG laser to ablate areas of endocardial scar to which earliest activation was documented in any given morphology of VT.

Unlike previous investigators, they have chosen to work on the beating normothermic heart during induced VT, persisting with laser photocoagulation until the particular VT stops. Heavy reliance is placed on detailed mapping, and this is reflected in prolonged pump times. However, the ischemic insult of aortic cross clamping is avoided, and there has been general improvement in ejection fraction; one patient died in surgery, and only one, with diffuse myocardial sarcoidosis, had inducible VT postoperatively. This is an interesting and appropriate new technology that deserves further application. If the initial enthusiastic reports are confirmed, the laser will assume an important role in VT ablation at operation.

The Automatic Implantable Cardioverter-Defibrillator (AICD)

An awareness of the high intensity of personnel and equipment needs for out-of-hospital cardiopulmonary resuscitation, including cardioversion for ventricular arrhythmia, provided motivation for the development of an implantable, fully automatic defibrillator, first reported some 15 years ago by Mirowsky et al.[81] After a decade of research and development, the device entered clinical testing, has subsequently been approved by the FDA, and is currently in clinical use.[82, 83] Originally designed as a defibrillating device, the current generation AICD identifies and treats VTs as well.

The device consists of a pulse generator and a set of three electrode leads. The pulse generator is quite large, weighs 292 gm, and is housed in a titanium case that contains the electronic components and the batteries. There are several configurations these electrodes may take, depending on the overall clinical condition. As originally designed, a defibrillating patch electrode was applied to the surface of the heart and a spring coil electrode was placed transvenously in the superior vena cava. The defibrillating electrode was designed to sense the configuration of the cardiac electrogram. The third lead was a bipolar catheter wedged in the apex of the right ventricle, for the purpose of sensing the heart rate and synchronizing the discharge with the R wave. If the chest is open, two epicardial screw-in electrodes can be substituted for the right ventricular lead.

The AICD continuously monitors the heart rate as well as the waveform configuration. The device is programmed to discharge when the heart rate exceeds a cutoff level and/or the cardiac electrogram has spent a critical time at or near the isoelectric line; the capacitor is discharged when the stored charge reaches approximately 720 V, and a shock of 25 joules is delivered approximately 17 seconds after the onset of arrhythmia. In the presence of VT, the discharge is programmed to be synchronous with the R wave. If the initial discharge does not convert the tachycardia, an additional pulse of 30 joules will be delivered three additional times. The pulse generator can be activated and deactivated by a magnet and can be interrogated in a systematic way to determine the integrity of the sensing function, the degree of battery depletion, and the number of pulses delivered to the patient.

Patient Selection

Patients who are at high risk of sudden death from malignant and refractory ventricular arrhythmia are suitable candidates for the device if corrective surgery is not feasible. The patient population must be thoroughly studied with PES and characterized as having inducible VT despite drug therapy. Additionally, in patients undergoing an antiarrhythmia operation, a defibrillating patch may be placed on the epicardial surface if the operation is considered by the surgeon to be less than ideal. Then, if inducibility persists subsequently despite drug therapy, the remaining two leads can be placed pervenously and the AICD can be implanted at that time.

Surgical Approaches

The exact surgical approach is determined by clinical circumstances. Although subxiphoid and subcostal approaches to the left ventricle may be utilized for placement of the single defibrillating patch, to be supplemented with pervenous electrodes as described above, there is better potential for more precise application via median sternotomy. This approach, of course, is appropriate when other cardiac procedures are being performed. Evidence is emerging that function of the device may be improved somewhat if two epicardial patches are utilized rather than one, obviating the need for a superior vena cava coil electrode; a bipolar screw-in system can be utilized for sensing and timing the discharge. This median sternotomy and double patch technique has become a preferred approach for several groups. If the patient has undergone previous surgery, particularly recently, a limited left-sided thoracotomy may be chosen, and the epicardial patch lead may be placed outside the pericardium, where it functions just as well as when directly on the epicardial surface.

The usual surgical complications associated with implanting a large device apply here: infection, hemorrhage, fluid accumulation around the pulse generator, and pericarditis; catheter perforation of the heart as well as displacement of the venous coil electrode have been reported. Malfunction due to random component failure and to loss of hermeticity have occurred rarely. False-positive discharges are less a problem now than in earlier models, where spurious signals due to lead fracture miscounted the heart rate, causing oversensing and subsequent discharge. Today, oversensing can still occur, particularly with fast supraventricular arrhythmias, and nonsustained VT may also trigger discharge during subsequent sinus rhythm. It is important to emphasize that drug therapy must be combined with use of the AICD in many instances, to control sinus rhythm and to suppress arrhythmias as far as possible. Subjective reactions of the patient to the internal discharges may vary from an almost complete lack of perceptible sensation to a very painful one. Most patients with implants that have discharged describe it as a moderate blow to the chest, "a kick from the inside" resulting in momentary discomfort. Serious and disabling emotional reactions have been recorded, however, particularly in patients who have received many shocks in a short time. If this occurs the device should be deactivated, and further diagnostic and rhythm control measures can be exercised in an intensive care setting.

Results

Data have been carefully gathered and analyzed for several years during clinical trials before FDA approval, over 300 cases having been done, primarily at Johns Hopkins Hospital, Baltimore, and Stanford (Calif.) University. With the original defibrillating device, the 1-year arrhythmic mortality was 11% in 37 patients.[83] As the device has evolved into the currently available AICD, the arrhythmic mortality has dropped markedly, to 1.9% in 209 patients.[84] In this population, the expected mortality ranges between 30% and 66% per year, putting into perspective the remarkable track record of this sophisticated device. Under current testing is a new generation of AICDs that will be programmed to terminate VT by means of overdrive or burst pacing.

Pacing

The stimulus for the use of ventricular overdrive pacing to terminate VT is the knowledge that many such arrhythmias can reproducibly be converted to sinus rhythm with programmed stimulation.[85, 86] After exhaustive electrophysiologic study, an antitachycardia pacemaker can be placed and programmed to terminate VT according to rate detection criteria.[87] Permanently implanted devices capable of both burst pacing and programmed overdrive pacing are available. This technology is now being incorporated into the AICD. Once this capability for countershock, and for overdrive and burst pacing, is incorporated into a single implantable device, it will be problematic whether placement of devices lacking the defibrillation feature will be justifiable, given the tendency of arrhythmia characteristics to change with time. It must be emphasized that these technologies, sophisticated as they may be, should be limited in their use to patients in whom curative surgery is not feasible.

Catheter Ablation

The use of high-energy intracardiac direct current shock for attempted ablation of postinfarction arrhythmogenic sources within the left ventricle has its background in animal and human studies directed toward ablation of the His bundle.[88, 89] After extensive endocardial mapping and location of right ventricular outflow tract and septal sources of tachycardia, Hartzler,[90] using general anesthesia, applied 300-joule shocks through the tip electrode of a standard 7 F quadripolar electrode catheter positioned adjacent to the site of earliest endocardial activation. The discharges were directed toward a paddle applied to the back, lateral chest wall, and anterior chest wall. Three patients were reported as being successfully treated, although one required a repeated treatment, which resulted in complete heart block, the need for a permanent pacemaker, and eventual death from severe biventricular failure. This technique has not become widely used, perhaps because a minority of patients have localized foci of origin and large areas of scar over which arrhythmias can be generated and travel. Further development of this concept is clearly indicated, but at present it must be considered experimental.[91, 92]

Conclusions and Future Directions

The use of indirect and incomplete surgical methods for the control of VT and VF can no longer be justified. This includes such methods as sympathectomy (with certain caveats), myocardial revascularization alone or with simple ventricular aneurysmectomy, and even limited epicardially based incisions or excisions in areas suspected or delineated by mapping as being a source or a pathway for the propagation of VT. The indicated surgical approach must ideally follow a period of investigation, if time permits, that utilizes the full array of electrophysiologic diagnostic methods fully to characterize the conduction system and its aberrancies. In individual cases where there is no coexisting obvious indication for surgery, the goal is to achieve accurate electrophysiologic diagnosis with a view toward selection of antiarrhythmia therapy by specific drug(s) that prevents inducibility of VT/VF using PES. In the rare situation in which incessant VT exists, is hemodynamically compromising, and does not allow a systematic approach, a reasonably complete operation can be done with or without the guidance of intraoperative mapping. However, in the usual setting, most patients come to operation after failure of drug treatment or the failure to find a drug that renders VT noninducible.

The surgical team, which includes a cardiologist-electrophysiologist and their support group, as well as the surgeon and his support group, currently has a choice of three methods of ablation: resection of endocardial scar tissue, application of cryolesions, and laser ablation. These methods may legitimately be applied in a variety of settings vis-à-vis electrophysiologic diagnosis, both preoperatively and intraoperatively. Ideally, surgery should be undertaken after thorough right and left ventricular catheter mapping, designed to localize the site(s) of earliest activation. These findings should be confirmed at surgery for all morphologies of VT, either spontaneous or induced, including any new morphologies discovered at the time of operation. In truth, this ideal is achieved only sporadically in most institutions doing antiarrhythmia surgery. The practicalities of dealing with the surgery of arrhythmia often countermand thorough PES and drug trials. Detailed preoperative endocardial mapping may not be chosen or may not be feasible in any individual case: the literature on mapping vs. visually guided endocardial ablation does not establish a clear advantage of endocardial mapping. Resection of all endocardial scar with or without cryolesions or laser ablation can be justified when complete study preoperatively is not feasible or warranted. Thus, at present, the four main categories of operative approach are limited endocardial resection that is map guided; complete resection of all visible endocardial scar with or without additional map guidance; cryolesions, which may be utilized as the sole means of ablation or in conjunction with endocardial resection of scar; and finally, laser ablation, which may be utilized alone or in combination with other methods, assuming that the early reports of its effectiveness are confirmed by other workers.

The various antiarrhythmia procedures have an operative mortality that clusters around 10% and will be difficult to lower further because of the nature and stage of disease in this patient cohort. All surviving patients should be studied with PES before hospital discharge to assess inducibility and to guide drug therapy if it is necessary to prevent inducibility. The inducibility rate following a thorough, carefully done surgical procedure should be 10% or less. The ensuing mortality, which is appreciable, should be due primarily to cardiac causes other than arrhythmia, and this is borne out by long-term follow-up studies; 5-year survival data indicate that 10% to 15% of a 30% to 35% attrition rate is from arrhythmia. When one considers that the 1-year mortality in this substrate of patients is 30% to 66% per year if treated by drugs alone, the attrition rate after surgery seems less forbidding.

As the AICD enters widespread clinical use, it is apparent that this sophisticated technology has been highly effective. The device can be used as a primary antiarrhythmia treatment, although nearly always supplemented with drug therapy, or as a supplemental measure secondary to antiarrhythmia surgery. The disadvantages are a respectably low incidence of component failure, the usual complications associated with large implanted foreign bodies, and the need for generator replacement approximately every 36 months.

To further improve the results of surgery for arrhythmia will be increasingly difficult in view of the dramatic strides made during the past decade. However, further development in several areas should eventually allow for further improvement in quality of life for victims of VT/VF. Appropriately aggressive surgical therapy and continued use of laser ablation should improve the arrhythmia-free survival beyond the current 80% level at 5 years. The early efforts at computer-assisted mapping and the use of various devices with numerous electrode pairs that can obtain simultaneous electrograms from epicardium and/or endocardium should allow more rapid and precise mapping at the time of operation and should provide data that will add further to our knowledge about the generation and transmission of VT.[93–95] This should in turn suggest the development of improved surgical procedures. Further development of pacing technology designed to control arrhythmias continues. The combination of defibrillating and overdrive-burst pacing will soon be available; as the device is further miniaturized, and with improved internal components, this technology will become even more acceptable and more widely applied. Thus, although postinfarction ventricular arrhythmias will always be life-threatening and frightening to the individual, their management should gradually become more routine and the overall results of treatment more satisfactory.

References

1. Lewis T, Rothschild MA: The excitatory process in the dog's heart: II. The ventricles. *Philos Trans R Soc Lond* 1915; 206:181–226.
2. Barker PS, Macleod AG, Alexander J: The excitatory process observed in the exposed human heart. *Am Heart J* 1930; 5:720–742.
3. Durrer D, VanDam RT, Freud GE, et al: Total excitation of the isolated human heart. *Circulation* 1970; 41:899–912.
4. Wellens HJJ: Pathophysiology of ventricular tachycardia in man. *Arch Intern Med* 1975; 135:473–479.
5. Durrer D, VanLier AAW, Buller J: Epicardial and intramural excitation in chronic myocardial infarction. *Am Heart J* 1964; 68:765–772.
6. Kaiser GA, Waldo AL, Harris PD, et al: New method to delineate myocardial damage at surgery. *Circulation* 1969; 39,40(suppl 1):83–89.
7. Kastor JA, Spear JF, Moore EN: Localization of ventricular irritability by epicardial mapping. *Circulation* 1972; 45:952–964.
8. Fontaine G, Frank R, Guiraudon G: Surgical treatment of resistant ventricular tachycardia by ventriculotomy: A new application of epicardial mapping. *Circulation* 1974; 319(suppl):49–50.
9. Wu D, Ammat-y-Leon F, Simpson RJ, et al: Electrophysiologic studies with multiple drugs in patients with A-V reentrant tachycardias utilizing an extranodal pathway. *Circulation* 1977; 56:727.
10. Horowitz LN, Josephson ME, Farshidi A, et al: Recurrent sustained ventricular tachycardia: Role of the electrophysiologic study in selection of antiarrhythmic regimens. *Circulation* 1978; 58:971.
11. Horowitz LN, Josephson ME, Kastor J: Intracardiac electrophysiologic studies as a method for optimization of drug therapy in chronic ventricular arrhythmia, in Sonnenblick E, (ed): *Sudden Cardiac Death,* ed 3. New York, Grune & Stratton, 1978, pp 251–268.
12. Uhl HS: A previously undescribed malformation of the heart: Almost total absence of the myocardium of the right ventricle. *Bull Johns Hopkins Hosp* 1956; 91:197.
13. Guiraudon G, Fontaine G, Frank R, et al: Surgical treatment of ventricular tachycardia guided by ventricular mapping in 23 patients without coronary artery disease. *Ann Thorac Surg* 1981; 32:439–450.
14. Moran JM, Kehoe RF, Loeb JM, et al: Operative therapy of malignant ventricular rhythm disturbances. *Ann Surg* 1983; 198:479–486.
15. Jervell A, Lang-Nielson F: Congenital deaf-mutism, functional heart disease with prolongation of the Q-T interval, and sudden death. *Am Heart J* 1957; 54:59
16. James TN, Froggatt P, Atkinson WJ Jr, et al: De subitaneis mortibus XXX: Observation on the pathophysiology of the long Q-T syndromes with special reference to the neuropathology of the heart. *Circulation* 1978; 57:1221.
17. Schwartz PJ, Periti M, Malliani A: The long Q-T syndrome. *Clin Cardiol* 1975; 89:378.
18. Moss AJ, McDonald J: Unilateral cervicothoracic sympathetic ganglionectomy for the treatment of long Q-T syndrome. *N Engl J Med* 1971; 285:903.
19. Schaffer WA, Cobb LA: Recurrent ventricular fibrillation and modes of death in survivors of out-of-hospital ventricular fibrillation. *N Engl J Med* 1975; 293:259–262.

20. Kehoe R, Moran JM, Zheutlin T, et al: Invasive electrophysiologic study to direct therapy in survivors of pre-hospital ventricular fibrillation. *Am J Cardiol* 1982; 49:928.
21. Ruskin J, DiMarco J, Garan H: Out-of-hospital cardiac arrest: Electrophysiologic observations and selection of long-term anti-arrhythmic therapy. *N Engl J Med* 1980; 303:607–613.
22. LeRiche R, Fontaine R: Chirurgie du Sympathique. *Rev Neurol* 1929; 1:1046.
23. White JC, Smithwick RH, Simeone FA: *The Autonomic Nervous System.* New York, Macmillan Publishing Co, 1952, p 288.
24. Harris AS, Estandia A, Tillotson RF: Ventricular ectopic rhythms and ventricular fibrillation following cardiac sympathectomy and coronary occlusion. *Am J Physiol* 1951; 165:505–515.
25. Estes EH Jr, Izlas HL Jr: Recurrent ventricular tachycardia: A case successfully treated by bilateral cardiac sympathectomy. *Am J Med* 1961; 31:493.
26. Zipes DP, Festoff B, Schaal SF, et al: Treatment of ventricular arrhythmia by permanent atrial pacemaker and cardiac sympathectomy. *Ann Intern Med* 1968; 68:591.
27. Nitter-Hauge S, Storstein O: Surgical treatment of recurrent ventricular tachycardia. *Br Heart J* 1973; 35:1132.
28. Couch OA Jr: Cardiac aneurysm with ventricular tachycardia and subsequent excision of aneurysm. *Circulation* 1959; 20:251.
29. Likoff W, Bailey CP: Problem of myocardial aneurysm: Recognition and treatment. *Circulation* 1956; 14:968.
30. Parkinson J, Bedford DE, Thompson WAR: Cardiac aneurysm. *Q J Med* 1938; 7:455.
31. Loop FD, Effler DB, Navia JA, et al: Aneurysms of the left ventricle: Survival and results of a 10-year surgical experience, 400 patients. *Ann Surg* 1973; 178:399.
32. Moran JM, Scanlon PJ, Nemickas R, et al: Surgical treatment of postinfarction ventricular aneurysm. *Ann Thorac Surg* 1976; 21:107.
33. Hunt D, Sloman G, Westlake G: Ventricular aneurysmectomy for recurrent tachycardia. *Br Heart J* 1969; 31:264–266.
34. Ritter ER: Intractable ventricular tachycardia due to ventricular aneurysm with surgical cure. *Ann Intern Med* 1969; 71:1155–1157.
35. Rolette E, Webster S, Avioli LF: Surgical management of ventricular aneurysm. *JAMA* 1969; 210:122–125.
36. Wardekar A, Lon B, Gosaynie CD, et al: Recurrent ventricular tachycardia successfully treated by excision of ventricular aneurysm. *Chest* 1972; 62:505–508.
37. Thind GS, Blakemore WS, Zinsser HF: Ventricular aneurysmectomy for the treatment of recurrent ventricular tachycardia. *Am J Cardiol* 1971; 27:690–694.
38. Magidson O: Resection of postmyocardial infarction ventricular aneurysms for cardiac arrhythmias. *Dis Chest* 1969; 56:211.
39. Maloy WC, Arrants JEE, Sorrell BF, et al: Left ventricular aneurysm of uncertain etiology with recurrent ventricular arrhythmias. *N Engl J Med* 1971; 285:662.
40. Ecker RE, Mullins CB, Grammer JC, et al: Control of intractable ventricular tachycardia by coronary revascularization. *Circulation* 1971; 44:666–671.
41. Nakhjavan EK, Morse DP, Nichols HT, et al: Emergency aortocoronary bypass: Treatment of ventricular tachycardia due to ischemic heart disease. *JAMA* 1971; 216:2138–2140.

42. Boineau JP, Cox JL: Rationale for a direct surgical approach to control ventricular arrhythmias. Am J Cardiol 1982; 49:381.
43. Kaiser GA, Ghahramani A, Bolooki H, et al: Role of coronary artery surgery in patients surviving unexpected cardiac arrest. Surgery 1975; 78:749.
44. Graham AF, Miller DC, Stinson EB, et al: Surgical treatment of refractory life-threatening ventricular tachycardia. Am J Cardiol 1973; 32:909–912.
45. Kenaan G, Mendez AM, Zubiate P, et al: Surgery for ventricular tachycardia unresponsive to medical treatment. Chest 1973; 64:574.
46. Mundth ED, Buckley JM, DeSanctis RW, et al: Surgical treatment of ventricular irritability. J Thorac Cardiovasc Surg 1973; 66:943.
47. Moran JM, Talano JV, Euler D: Refractory ventricular arrhythmia: The role of intraoperative electrophysiological study. Surgery 1977; 82:809–815.
48. Spurrell RAJ, Sowton E, Deuchar DC: Ventricular tachycardia in four patients evaluated by programmed electrical stimulation of the heart and treated in two patients by surgical division of the anterior radiation of left bundle branch. Br Heart J 1973; 35:1014.
49. Spurrell RAJ, Yates AK, Thorburn CW, et al: Surgical treatment of ventricular tachycardia after epicardial mapping studies. Br Heart J 1975; 37:115.
50. Wittig JH, Boineau JP: Surgical treatment of ventricular arrhythmias using epicardial, transmural, and endocardial mapping. Ann Thorac Surg 1975; 20:117–126.
51. Guiraudon G, Fontaine G, Frank R, et al: Encircling endocardial ventriculotomy: A new surgical treatment for life-threatening ventricular tachycardias resistant to medical treatment following myocardial infarction. Ann Thorac Surg 1978; 26:438–444.
52. Harken AH, Josephson ME, Horowitz LN: Surgical endocardial resection for the treatment of malignant ventricular tachycardia. Ann Surg 1979; 190:456–460.
53. Moran JM, Kehoe RF, Loeb JM, et al: Extended endocardial resection for the treatment of ventricular tachycardia and ventricular fibrillation. Ann Thorac Surg 1982; 34:538–552.
54. Camm H, Ward ED, Spurrell RAJ, et al: Cryothermal mapping and cryoablation in the treatment of refractory cardiac arrhythmias. Circulation 1980; 62:67.
55. Gallagher JJ, Anderson RW, Kasell J, et al: Cryoablation of drug-resistant ventricular tachycardia in a patient with a variant of scleroderma. Circulation 1978; 57:190.
56. Mason JW, Stinson EB, Oyer PE, et al: Mapping guided surgical therapy of refractory ventricular tachycardia due to coronary artery disease, abstracted. Am J Cardiol 1983; 49:947.
57. Guiraudon GM, Klein GJ, Jones DL, et al: Encircling endocardial cryoablation for ventricular arrhythmias after myocardial infarction: Further experience. Circulation 1985; 72(suppl 3):222.
58. Mesnildry P, Laborde F, Piwnica A, et al: Encircling thermo-exclusion by the Nd-YAG laser without mapping: A new surgical technique for ischemic ventricular tachycardia, abstracted. Circulation 1985; 72(suppl 3):389.
59. Selle JG, Svenson RH, Sealy WC, et al: Successful clinical laser ablation of ventricular tachycardia: A promising new therapeutic method. Ann Thorac Surg 1986; 42:380–384.
60. Loeb JM, Whitson CC, Kehoe RF, et al: Facilitation of endocardial mapping during ventricular tachycardia. Circulation 1981; 64:88.

61. Moran JM, Kehoe RF, Loeb JM, et al: The role of papillary muscle resection and mitral valve replacement in the control of refractory ventricular arrhythmia. *Circulation* 1983; 68 (suppl 2):154–160.
62. Cox JL: Surgery for cardiac arrhythmias. *Curr Probl Cardiol* 1983; 8:48–55.
63. Landymore R: Personal communication, February 9, 1987.
64. Ungerleider RM, Holman WL, Stanley TE, et al: Encircling endocardial ventriculotomy for refractory ischemic ventricular tachycardia: I. Electrophysiologic effects. *J Thorac Cardiovasc Surg* 1982; 83:840.
65. Ungerleider RM, Holman WL, Stanley TE, et al: Encircling endocardial ventriculotomy for refractory ischemic ventricular tachycardia: II. Effects on regional myocardial blood flow. *J Thorac Cardiovasc Surg* 1982; 83:850.
66. Ungerleider RM, Holman WL, Calcagno D, et al: Encircling endocardial ventriculotomy for refractory ischemic ventricular tachycardia: III. Effects on regional left ventricular function. *J Thorac Cardiovasc Surg* 1982; 83:857.
67. Cox JL, Gallagher JJ, Ungerleider RM: Encircling endocardial ventriculotomy for refractory ischemic ventricular tachycardia: IV. Clinical indications, surgical technique, mechanism of action, and surgical results. *J Thorac Cardiovasc Surg* 1982; 83:865.
68. Harken A, Josephson M: Recurrent ventricular tachycardia: How effective is surgical management? *Am J Surg* 1983; 145:718.
69. Brodman R, Fisher JD, Johnston DR, et al: Results of electro-physiologically guided operations for drug-resistant recurrent ventricular tachycardia and ventricular fibrillation due to coronary artery disease. *J Thorac Cardiovasc Surg* 1984; 87:431–438.
70. Mason JW, Stinson EB, Oyer PE: Arrhythmia mechanisms and outcome in surgery for recurrent ventricular tachycardia. *Circulation* 1983; 68(suppl 3):176.
71. Borggrefe M, Breithardt G, Ostermeyer J: Partial endocardial encircling ventriculotomy for drug-refractory ventricular tachycardia associated with ischemic heart disease. *Circulation* 1985; 72(suppl 3):221.
72. Anderson KP, Mason JW: Surgical management of ventricular tachy-arrhythmias. *Clin Cardiol* 1983; 6:415–425.
73. Kehoe R, Zheutlin T, Finkelmeier, et al: Visually directed endo-cardial resection for ventricular arrhythmia: Long-term outcome and functional status. *J Am Coll Cardiol* 1985; 5(suppl 2):497.
74. Moran JM, Kehoe RF, Spies S: Extended endocardial resection for treatment of ventricular arrhythmia: Effect on LV function. *Circulation* 1983; 68(suppl 3):116.
75. Lawrie GM, Wyndham CRC, Krafchek J: Progress in the surgical treatment of cardiac arrhythmias. *JAMA* 1985; 254:1464–1468.
76. Landymore RW, Kinley CE, Gardner M: Encircling endocardial resection with complete removal of endocardial scar without intra-operative mapping for the ablation of drug-resistant ventricular tachycardia. *J Thorac Cardiovasc Surg* 1985; 89:18–24.
77. Harrison L, Gallagher JJ, Kassel J, et al: Cryosurgical ablation of the A-V node-His bundle: A new method for producing A-V block. *Circulation* 1977; 55:463.
78. Gallagher JJ, Anderson RW, Kasell J, et al: Cryoablation of drug-resistant ventricular tachycardia in a patient with a variant of scleroderma. *Circulation* 1978; 57:190–197.

79. Cox JL: Anatomic-electrophysiologic basis for the surgical treatment of refractory ischemic ventricular tachycardia. *Ann Surg* 1983; 198:119.
80. Wyndham CR, Krafchek J, Lawrie GM: Cryoablation of ventricular tachycardia in the interventricular septum: Initial experience with a new biventricular approach. *Circulation* 1985; 72(suppl 3):221.
81. Mirowski M, Mower MM, Staewen WS, et al: Standby automatic defibrillator: An approach to prevention of sudden coronary death. *Arch Intern Med* 1970; 126:158.
82. Mirowski M, Reid PR, Mower MM, et al: Termination of malignant ventricular arrhythmias with an implanted automatic defibrillator in human beings. *N Engl J Med* 1980; 303:322.
83. Watkins L Jr, Mirowski M, Mower MM, et al: Automatic defibrillation in man: The initial surgical experience. *J Thorac Cardiovasc Surg* 1981; 82:492.
84. Mirowski M: The automatic implantable cardioverter-defibrillator: An overview. *J Am Coll Cardiol* 1985; 6:461–466.
85. Johnson RA, Hutter AM, DeSanctis RW, et al: Chronic overdrive pacing in the control of refractory ventricular arrhythmias. *Ann Intern Med* 1974; 80:380–383.
86. Cooper TB, Maclean WAH, Waldo AL: Overdrive pacing for supra-ventricular tachycardia: A review of theoretical implications and therapeutic techniques. *PACE* 1978; 1:196–221.
87. Griffin JC, Mason JW, Calfee RV: The treatment of ventricular tachycardia using an automatic tachycardia terminating pacemaker. *PACE* 1981; 4:582–588.
88. Scheinman MM, Morady F, Hess DS, et al: Catheter-induced ablation of the atrioventricular junction to control refractory supraventricular arrhythmias. *JAMA* 1982; 248:851–855.
89. Gallagher JJ, Svenson RH, Kasell JH, et al: Catheter technique for closed-chest ablation of the atrioventricular conduction system. *N Engl J Med* 1982; 306:194–200.
90. Hartzler GO: Electrode catheter ablation of refractory focal ventricular tachycardia. *J Am Coll Cardiol* 1983; 2:1107–1113.
91. Scheinman MM, Davis JC: Catheter ablation for treatment of tachy-arrhythmias: Present role and potential promise. *Circulation* 1986; 73:10–13.
92. Tonet JL, Fontaine G, Frank R, et al: Treatment of refractory ventricular tachycardias by endocardial fulguration. *Circulation* 1985; 72(suppl 3):388.
93. Ideker RE, Smith WM, Wallace AG, et al: A computerized method for the rapid display of ventricular activation during the intra-operative study of arrhythmias. *Circulation* 1979; 59:449.
94. Mickleborough LL, Harris L, Downar E, et al: A new approach for mapping ventricular tachycardia (VT), abstracted. *Circulation* 1985; 72(suppl 3):222.
95. Fann JI, Loeb JM, LoCicero J III, et al: Endocardial activation mapping and endocardial pace-mapping using a balloon apparatus. *Am J Cardiol* 1985; 55:1076–1083.

Calcium and the Myocardium: Physiologic and Pathologic Processes

Glenn A. Langer, M.D.

Professor of Medicine and Physiology, Castera Professor of Cardiology, Associate Dean for Research, UCLA School of Medicine, Los Angeles, California

The mammalian heart modulates its force development by the use of just two general mechanisms: (1) the Frank-Starling response to changing preload, which involves a change in diastolic fiber length; (2) a change of contractile state in which force changes without a primary change in diastolic fiber length. The first mechanism involves a primary change in the relation of sarcomeric myofilaments to each other. There is increasing evidence[1] that length changes associated with variation in preload also induce changes in intracellular calcium distribution and/or myofilament sensitivity that may affect force, but the primary event remains the length change. The second mechanism, change in contractile state, primarily depends on alterations in cellular Ca flux and exchange, and this chapter will focus on this subject.

Before discussing the force-related movements of Ca, it is necessary to review, briefly, the pertinent ultrastructure of the myocardial cell, emphasizing those structures believed to be of most importance in the control of Ca movement.

Ultrastructure

Figure 1 includes most of the organelles to be discussed.

Cellular Surface

The first cellular structure that is encountered as one proceeds from the interstitium is the *glycocalyx*.[2] This structure is composed of glycoproteins, glycolipids, and free polysaccharides. It has two components: an outer layer or external lamina (30 nm) and an inner layer or surface coat (20 nm). The surface coat component is an inherent part of the sarcolemma (SL; see later). The glycocalyx contains a large number of negatively charged moieties and does, therefore, bind Ca. In fact, in the absence of Ca (<25 μM $[Ca]_o$, or extracellular concentration of Ca), the external lam-

Adv Card Surg 1:55–75, 1990

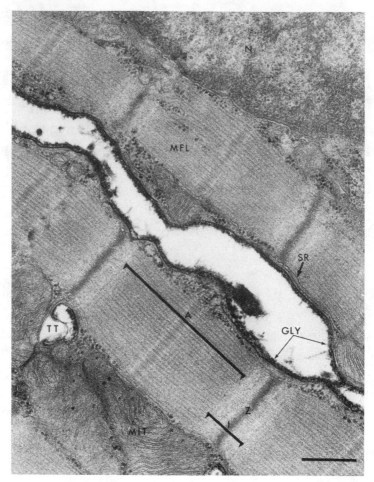

FIG 1.
Electron micrograph of portions of two myocardial cells. N = nucleus; MFL = myofilaments; SR = a component of junctional (subsarcolemmal) sarcoplasmic reticulum; GLY = glycocalyx; Z = Z line of sarcomere; I = I band of sarcomere; A = A band of sarcomere; TT = transverse tubule cut in cross section; MIT = mitochondria. The clear area bordered by GLY is the interstitial space between the cells. The dark line under the GLY is the sarcolemmal lipid bilayer. The scale at bottom right represents 0.5 μm. (Courtesy of Dr. J. S. Frank.)

ina separates from the surface coat. This indicates that there is a Ca-dependent bridging between the components. The role of the glycocalyx with respect to the Ca exchange of the cell is not settled. It should be mentioned, however, that the removal of a major glycocalyx constituent, sialic acid, has a marked effect on Ca permeability.[3] It was found, using monolayers of myocardial cells in tissue culture, that specific removal of sialic acid (a negatively charged nine-carbon amino sugar) by the enzyme neuraminidase caused a many-fold increase in the cell's permeability to Ca without an effect on the cell's potassium permeability. This would indicate that the glycocalyx could play an important role in the control of basic Ca permeability of the cell. The structure has been somewhat neglected in examination, for example, of the effects of ischemia. Jennings et al.[4] did note, however, that ischemia is associated with separation of the glycocalyx components from the cell surface, and the possibility arises that this could contribute to the well-recognized Ca leak that develops during ischemia.

As one proceeds inward, deep to the surface coat lies the *lipid bilayer* (7.5 to 9.0 nm thick). The fundamental structure of the bilayer consists of two layers of phospholipid molecules, each with a fatty acid tail that is hydrophobic and a phosphate-containing head that is hydrophilic. Thus, these molecules are amphiphilic, with the hydrophobic tail oriented in the inner direction and the hydrophilic head oriented to the water in the interstitium (outer leaflet) or to the water in the cytoplasm (inner leaflet). Embedded within the lipid bilayer are intramembrane particles, 8 to 10 nm in diameter, that represent the membrane proteins and are the manifestation of channels and enzymes. This arrangement, with proteins distributed within the lipid, is now the universally accepted membrane model initially described as the "fluid mosaic" model by Singer and Nicolson.[5] Some of the proteins and lipids have sugars attached to them, and these components extend into the surface coat component of the glycocalyx. Therefore, the surface coat is an integral part of SL structure.

With respect to Ca, the bilayer phospholipids bind a large amount of the ion.[2] A fraction of the intramembrane proteins represent Ca channels, the sodium-Ca exchangers, and the SL Ca pump. The channel is a potential-sensitive system that allows entry of Ca to the cell during a portion of the action potential. The Na-Ca exchanger couples the movement of these ions across the bilayer and, depending on conditions, can produce net inward or outward Ca and Na flux. The SL Ca pump is an adenosine triphosphate (ATP)–dependent system capable of pumping Ca out of the cell. These three systems (channel, exchanger, and pump) are, at present, the only known pathways for Ca movement across the bilayer.

There are two variations of the surface membrane. At the level of the Z line of each sarcomere, the SL invaginates to form the transverse tubular system or *T system*. The glycocalyx also invaginates with the bilayer, so the T-system tubules contain glycocalyx material. The T tubules extend to the center of the cell and in some regions they assume an axial orientation parallel to the sarcomere. The effect of the T tubules is to bring the events taking place along the SL, as well as the content of the interstitial space, to the ends of each sarcomere of the cell. Since each sarcomere is approximately 2 μm long, and there is a T tubule at each end, the T-tubular membrane is, at most, 1 μm from every portion of the sarcomere. This makes the distance for diffusion of substances from the cellular surface, including Ca, quite small.

The second variation is at the points where the SL of two cells comes into apposition. This is where the *nexus* is formed. At this point the SL of the cells is separated by a 2-nm gap. The gap is bridged with particles with central open cores of about 2 nm that represent channels between cells.[6] These channels provide access to ion flow from cell to cell. The nexus is, then, a site of low-resistance coupling between cells and provides the pathway for electrical conduction from cell to cell.

Intracellular Components

The *sarcoplasmic reticulum* (SR) is an intracellular membranous structure critical to the control of Ca movement. The SR has two components: (1) the "longitudinal SR" is composed of approximately 25-nm tubules that wrap around the A and I bands of the sarcomere; (2) the "junctional SR" is the portion that comes into close contact with the peripheral or T-tubular SL. The two components are part of a continuous, interconnected system within the cell. It is generally accepted that the longitudinal SR contains the proteins that represent the Ca-pumping system responsible for the intracellular sequestration of Ca that is necessary to remove Ca from the myofilaments in order that relaxation be achieved. The Ca pumped by the longitudinal tubules moves into the junctional SR, believed to serve as the storage region. This Ca is that released to the myofilaments on excitation in order that contraction be initiated. The process of release from the junctional SR is clearly different in skeletal and cardiac muscle.[7, 8] Skeletal muscle contraction does not require the presence of extracellular Ca,[9] whereas cardiac muscle clearly does.[10] In skeletal muscle, the signal for release is believed to be either a transmitted electrical signal from the SL or the release of a chemical messenger (inositol triphosphate) after excitation. The question remains undecided. In heart muscle, evidence strongly favors the concept that the Ca that enters the cell across the SL on excitation induces a release of more Ca from the junctional SR[8] (Ca-induced Ca release).

The *mitochondria* occupy about 35% of cellular volume.[11] Their length varies between 2 and 8 μm, and, therefore, a single mitochondrion may span several of the approximately 2-μm-long sarcomeres. Though the mitochondria have the capacity to take up Ca and release it, it is unlikely that they participate in the beat-to-beat control of Ca movement in the cell. They do become important, however, as a Ca-buffering system under conditions of high Ca loading such as may occur with reperfusion after a period of ischemia.

The last structural entity of importance in the relation of Ca to force control is the *myofibril structure*. This is the end point in the Ca-controlled process. The myofibrils occupy the largest fraction of cell volume, about 48%.[11] They are made up of myofilaments, thick and thin, arranged to produce the structure of the sarcomere. The thick filaments are composed largely of myosin and form the A band of the sarcomere. The thin filaments are anchored at the Z line of each sarcomere, and a set of thin filaments extends from each end of the sarcomere toward the center. The thin filaments are composed mainly of actin but contain other proteins important in Ca control, troponin and tropomyosin. The thin filaments form the I bands of the sarcomere. The thin filaments are arranged about thick filaments such that on cross section each thick filament is surrounded by six thin filaments over the region of the sarcomere where these filaments overlap. It is in this region of overlap of thick and thin filaments where force is generated by the heart muscle. Depending on the level of Ca about the troponin molecules attached to actin there will be attachment, through cross-bridge formation, of myosin to actin. This cross-bridge attachment and subsequent pulling of the actin filaments past myosin causes the sarcomere to shorten and generate force. Each muscle cell contains about 5,000 force-generating sarcomeres. The ventricles are composed of about 3 billion muscle cells. Thus, these pumping chambers contain some 1.5×10^{13} sarcomeric contractile units, all of which are coordinated to contribute to the total force developed with each cardiac cycle.

Figure 2 depicts, in schematic form, a segment of the cell in three dimensions. It shows the relationship of the T-tubular invaginations from the cellular surface occurring at the Z line register and the abutment of the lat-

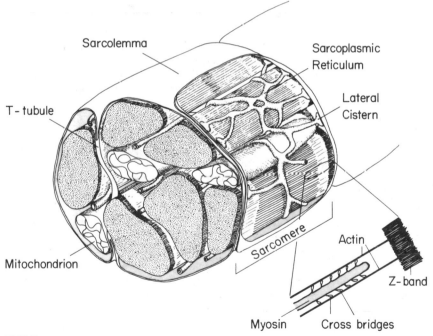

FIG 2.
Schematic of segment of a cardiac muscle cell with enlargement of portion of a myofibril to illustrate actin-myosin relationships. Sarcomere length is approximately 2 μm.

eral cisternae of the sarcoplasmic reticulum on the T-tube membrane. A segment of a sarcomere is enlarged, showing the actin filaments (thin filaments) anchored in the Z line. The actin filaments are oriented around a myosin filament (thick filament), with a set of the tension-generating crossbridges depicted.

Ca Movement

It has been recognized for many years that cardiac muscle requires the presence of Ca in the extracellular environment so that contraction can be maintained. A recently completed study[10] in isolated single myocardial cells clearly defines, on the basis of contractile function, two components of Ca: a "rapidly" exchangeable pool and a more "slowly" exchangeable pool. The rapid pool can be totally depleted and repleted in less than 1 second on removal and replenishment of extracellular Ca. Total depletion of this pool completely eliminates contraction. Force development is linearly related to the $[Ca]_o$ in this pool between 1.0 and 0mM. The Ca represented by this pool could simply be that in free solution in the interstitial space, but there is evidence that this is not the case.

SL Ca Binding

The curve that relates Ca binding to low-affinity sites in purified SL preparations at Ca concentrations from $50\mu M$ to 10mM and the curve that relates force development to $[Ca]_o$ over the same range of concentrations are superimposable.[12] The obvious conclusion is that there may be a quantitative relationship between SL Ca binding and force.

A series of other studies, recently reviewed,[13] support the importance of SL-bound Ca in force control. (1) The ability of a series of cations (lanthanum, cadmium, manganese, magnesium) to uncouple excitation from contraction is the same as their relative ability to displace Ca from SL. (2) Polymyxin B, the antibiotic, is a compound with a highly positively charged hydrophilic head and hydrophobic lipid tail. It specifically competes for Ca-binding sites on anionic and zwitterionic phospholipid of the SL. It is a potent displacer of Ca from cardiac cells and a potent uncoupler of excitation from contraction. (3) Phospholipase D (PLD) is an enzyme that specifically cleaves the nitrogenous base from SL phospholipid. This produces phosphatidic acid and thereby increases anionic hydrophilic groups. This increases Ca bound to the SL and increases force development of ventricular tissue. (4) Insertion of a negatively charged amphiphile (molecule with a hydrophobic and a hydrophilic end) into the SL increases Ca binding and force significantly. (5) Variation in pH produces significant effects on SL Ca binding that can be closely related to changes in contractile force.

The foregoing findings support the concept of a role for SL-bound Ca in contractile control. It seemed possible, however, that the interventions that produced changes in membrane charge (PLD, amphiphile insertion, Polymyxin B) also caused a change in the Ca in the so-called diffuse double layer. The diffuse double layer refers to the space (1 to 2 nm) directly adjacent to the SL where the ionic composition of the fluid in the space is a direct function of the membrane surface potential. For example, increase in negative charge in the membrane causes cationic movement, including Ca, into the diffuse double layer. Calcium in this region, rather than Ca actually bound to anionic SL sites, could conceivably be the component of rapidly exchangeable Ca important in contraction. This concept was examined with the use of a large cationic probe, dimethonium.[14] Dimethonium displaces cations, including Ca, from the diffuse double layer without affecting membrane-bound Ca.[15] Such displacement of Ca produces little or no effect on force development. Thus, it seems that it is the Ca actually bound to the SL, most likely to anionic phospholipid sites, that is an important component of the rapidly exchangeable pool.

Wherever the "external" Ca is located, it must be moved across the SL so that it may serve as the coupler between excitation and contraction. At present there are only two known paths by which Ca enters: (1) the Ca or so-called slow channel; (2) the Na-Ca exchanger.

Ca Channel

Current through a membrane channel is described by $I = \bar{g}(E_m - E_i)$, where $\bar{g}$ is the conductance for the ion carrying the current (I) and ($E_m - E_i$) is the difference between the transmembrane potential (E_m) at any instant and the equilibrium potential (E_i) for the ion under consideration. The equilibrium potential is that potential necessary to counteract exactly the movement of the ion down its concentration gradient across the cell membrane (the chemical "driving force") for the ion. The E_i is defined by the Nernst equation:

$$E_i = \frac{RT}{zF} \ln \frac{[X]_o}{[X]_i}$$

where R is gas constant, T is absolute temperature, F is Faraday (all constants at a particular temperature), z is valence of the ion, and $[X]_o$ and $[X]_i$ are the extracellular and intracellular concentrations of the ion, respectively. For Ca, E_i is approximately 80 to 120 mV, which is the E_m at which no net movement of Ca, in or out of the cell, will occur. In the course of an action potential, the trans-SL potential changes from -85 mV (rest) to $+20$ mV (peak depolarization) and back to rest. The intracellular Ca concentration, or $[Ca]_i$, also changes during the cardiac cycle from less than 10^{-7}M (rest) to about 5×10^{-6}M during peak contraction and back to the resting level. Thus, both the electrical and the chemical driving forces are continuously changing throughout the cycle. Since E_i for Ca is, however, strongly positive (80 to 120 mV), the driving force for the ion is always inward through the channel. It is more strongly inward at rest, when ($E_m - E_i$) is -180 to -160 mV, than at the peak of the action potential, when

$(E_m - E_i)$ is much less. However, even at the peak of the action potential (about 20 mV), the value of $(E_m - E_i)$ is still negative, and Ca would still show a net inward movement.

No matter the value of $(E_m - E_i)$, if $\bar{g}$ is zero or very low there will be little Ca movement. Such is the case at resting membrane potential, and not until the potential rises to -40 to -30 mV does $\bar{g}$ change. At this level, threshold voltage is reached and the Ca "gate" opens, $\bar{g}$ rises, and Ca moves according to the level of $(E_m - E_i)$ as described above. The Ca channel is, therefore, visualized to have a gating mechanism controlled by E_m. The gate remains open throughout the duration of the action potential plateau, or for some 150 to 200 msec, and Ca flows into the cell during this time. When the membrane potential falls below -30 to -40 mV, the gate closes, $\bar{g}$ falls, and Ca influx ceases.

In addition to the role of Ca in the coupling process of the ventricle, it plays a significant role in pacemaker tissue of the heart: the sinus and atrioventricular nodes. The slow Ca current has been identified as the primary inward current responsible for the action potential in both these tissues.[16, 17]

At present, the quantity of Ca that passes through the slow channel with each excitation is not known with any certainty. It is clear, however, that influx through the channel is absolutely necessary in order that contraction occur. Specific Ca-channel blockers (eg, the dihydropyridines such as nifedipine) are capable of completely abolishing contraction at a time when the slow inward current is abolished. Just as contraction and current can be abolished or decreased with the dihydropyridines, so can the reverse be achieved with small modification to the dihydropyridine molecule, which converts the antagonist to an agonist.[18] An example is Bay K 8644, which, when applied to cardiac tissue, binds to the Ca channel and augments both slow inward current and contraction.

The level of Ca conductance $(\bar{g}_{Ca})$ is the primary factor in the control of Ca influx. The likelihood that the Ca channel will be open above threshold depends on the degree to which the channel protein is phosphorylated. The basic effect fits the proposal of Kuo and Greengard[19, 20] that "regulation of protein kinases, leading to an altered state of phosphorylation of specific substrate protein, may be a general mechanism through which the diverse biologic effects of cyclic AMP are mediated." There is a cyclic adenosine monophosphate (AMP)–dependent protein kinase in the membrane that controls the degree of phosphorylation. The system accounts for the mechanism of catecholamine action.[21] Catechol stimulation of SL β-receptors stimulates adenyl cyclase, with subsequent augmentation of cyclic AMP levels. This leads to increased activation of the protein kinase and increased phosphorylation of the Ca-channel protein(s). This does not promote the addition of Ca channels but, as stated above, increases the likelihood of the channel remaining open over the period of activation, i.e., above threshold. The longer the channel remains open, the larger will be the integrated influx of Ca.

Parasympathetic stimulation is negatively inotropic. Ten Eick et al.,[22] using voltage clamp techniques, demonstrated that acetylcholine (ACh) reduced the slow inward current with coincident reduction in contractile force. George et al.[23] had previously shown that ACh increased levels of cyclic guanosine monophosphate (GMP), and increase of this compound is negatively inotropic.[24] Thus, parasympathetic stimulation initiates a series of events through the formation of cyclic GMP that is essentially opposite to those initiated by sympathetic stimulation.

The Na-Ca Exchanger

The other system capable of transport of Ca inward is the Na-Ca exchanger. It should be noted that, under physiologic conditions, this system probably operates to move Ca in a net outward direction. This notwithstanding, variations in the outward movement in the presence of stable inward flux will obviously result in changes in intracellular Ca level. Moreover, there seem to be certain conditions in which the exchanger would appear to account for net inward movement.

Work before 1964 focused on models of Na-Ca exchange in which the interaction between Na and Ca was considered to take place at the external surface of the cell, at which site Na and Ca ions would compete for anionic groups on a carrier that would subsequently move across the membrane.[25] In 1964, Repke,[26] in a consideration of the mechanism of action of digitalis, and Langer,[27] in a consideration of the force staircase response, raised the possibility that intracellular accumulation of Na might be linked to augmented Ca influx. In 1968, Reuter and Seitz[28] proposed a carrier system for Na and Ca and demonstrated that Ca efflux rate was sensitive to the concentration gradient for Na across the membrane. The following year, Baker et al.,[29] in a pivotal study, demonstrated in the internally perfused squid axon that Na and Ca movements were coupled in both directions, i.e., Na in−Ca out and Na out−Ca in. These studies all indicated a system more complex than binding to an anionic SL component and suggested the presence of an Na-Ca exchanger.

Initially it was believed that the coupling of the transport was in the ratio of $2:1$ (Na:Ca), an electroneutral process. However, Benninger et al.[30] pointed out that the free energy change (ΔF) required for movement of one Ca ion outward during diastole was much greater than the Δf for movement of two Na ions inward. Unless the coupling was greater than $2:1$ or there was another energy source, the exchanger would not work. It was soon shown that the coupling was not electroneutral but more likely to be $3:1$ (Na:Ca).[31]

The fact that the exchanger is charged means that its movement will be affected by the transmembrane potential. The exchanger will, then, have an equilibrium potential just as shown for a charged ion but will depend on the difference between the equilibrium potentials for the ions carried (Na and Ca) and the coupling ratio. Thus,

$$V_E = (nV_{Na} - 2V_{Ca})/(n - 2),$$

where V_E is equilibrium potential for the exchanger, n is coupling ratio ($3:1$), and V_{Na} and V_{Ca} are equilibrium potentials for Na and Ca, respectively (as defined by the Nernst relation previously described). In diastole,

V_{Na} is approximately 75 mV and V_{Ca} is about 120 mV. With n = 3, V_E = −15 mV. This means that at membrane potential more negative than −15 mV, the carrier would move Na inward and Ca outward; at membrane potentials more positive than −15 mV, the exchanger would move in the reverse direction, producing net movement of Ca inward. The estimation of exchanger movement during the course of the cardiac cycle is more complex, however.

As described for Ca movement through the channel, the equilibrium potential changes as $[Ca]_i$ changes. The $[Na]_i$ changes only slightly during a cycle, so E_{Na} remains essentially fixed. But as indicated, $[Ca]_i$ increases from 10^{-7} to 5×10^{-6} M for full activation. This will change V_{Ca} from 120 mV in diastole to 70 mV at peak contraction. This changes the equilibrium potential of the exchanger from −15 mV to +85 mV and indicates that the carrier will not reverse direction during the course of the action potential, i.e., it will continue to produce a net movement of Na inward and Ca outward. This does not mean, however, that interventions that affect exchanger movement could not play a role in augmentation of intracellular Ca.

It is not likely, in vivo, that significant changes in $[Na]_o$ or $[Ca]_o$ occur. Also, it is likely that steady-state $[Ca]_i$ will not vary beyond the range indicated during the course of the action potential. Steady-state $[Na]_i$, on the other hand, does vary in response to various interventions, e.g., change in stimulation frequency, digitalis administration.

The recent development of ion-selective microelectrodes (ISME) has permitted direct measurements of cellular Na activity (a^iNa) in the functional cell in various ventricular tissues. Stimulation produces a rate and time-dependent elevation of a^iNa as much as +30% for rapid rates.[32] As a^iNa increases, so does a^iCa associated with increased frequency of stimulation. The currently accepted explanation for this is as follows. An increase of heart rate increases cellular Na influx in proportion to the rate. For example, an increase from 60 to 120 beats per minute will essentially double Na influx per minute. Early studies[33] and the ISME studies noted above indicate that $[Na]_i$ increases as rate increases and remains at the higher level as long as the increased rate is maintained. The increase of $[Na]_i$ is due to "Na pump lag."[33] This lag occurs because the membrane Na-K pump regulates its pumping activity on the basis of the level of $[Na]_i$. On an increase in heart rate, the pump has to "wait" as a fraction of the increased Na influx is retained to provide the signal, i.e., increased $[Na]_i$, for increase of Na pumping. As the pump increases its activity, Na efflux again matches Na influx and a new steady-state, but higher, level of $[Na]_i$ is maintained. The new level represents a gain of only 2 to 3 mM in a^iNa, but this represents an increase of 30% or more (see above). This results in an increase in the $[Na]_i/[Na]_o$ ratio to which the Na-Ca exchanger is sensitive and results in a fall in Ca efflux and, perhaps, a rise in Ca influx. The net effect is to produce a rise in $[Ca]_i$, which accounts for the positive inotropic effect of an increase in stimulation frequency or the so-called "staircase effect."

The basic mechanism discussed with respect to the staircase explains the inotropic action of digitalis, not understood until almost 200 years after its description by William Withering.[34] The original concept was proposed by Repke[26] and further developed by Langer.[35] The primary action of the digitalis glycosides is inhibition of SL Na-K ATPase, the enzyme that controls the Na pump. This inhibition leads to an increase of $[Na]_i$.[36] Contractile force increases as a^iNa increases and is consistent with the expected effect on the Na-Ca exchanger, i.e., increase net Ca uptake by the cell. Digitalis induces an Na pump lag at fixed stimulation rate by inhibition of the Na pump. The discovery of the Na-Ca exchanger linked the primary effects of digitalis on the Na-K pump to the positive inotropic effect by providing the mechanism for increased intracellular Ca.

SL Ca Pump

There is one other system at the SL that is involved in Ca movement. The system operates to promote Ca efflux from the cell and was documented in 1980.[37] The system is ATP dependent and pumps 1 Ca for each mole of ATP hydrolyzed—half as efficient as the SR Ca pump. The SL Ca pump has a very high Ca affinity, with a K_m (half activation) of less than 1 μM. This indicates that it may function to maintain low intracellular levels of Ca during diastole. It is markedly responsive to calmodulin. Compared with the Na-Ca exchanger, the SL pump is much slower. The rapid exchanger may respond during the course of the action potential, leaving the SL pump to "mop up" during the diastolic period.

The discussion thus far has focused on Ca movement at the SL. We now move intracellularly.

SR

This organelle is responsible both for uptake and release of Ca. Calcium uptake across the SR membrane is mediated by a Ca:Mg–ATPase using ATP as a source of energy. Two Ca and one ATP bind to the external surface of the ATPase, ATP is hydrolyzed, and a high-energy phosphorylated compound is formed. Dephosphorylation occurs after the Ca is moved to the inner surface, and this releases Ca into the lumen. These events are believed to occur primarily in the longitudinal components of the SR. The system is stimulated by a cyclic AMP.[38] This cyclic nucleotide acts on a protein kinase to induce phosphorylation of a compound called *phospholamban*,[39] which, in the phosphorylated state, increases the activity of the Ca pump. It is possible that the well-recognized stimulation of the SR Ca pump by catecholamine is mediated through cyclic AMP–dependent protein kinase and phospholamban phosphorylation. The system can also be stimulated by calmodulin. The K_m of this system for Ca pumping is 1 to 2 μm. As $[Ca]_i$ rises during activation of contraction, the pump is activated and maximally stimulated as Ca reaches peak levels during systole. As Ca influx through the SL channel is shut off, the SR pump actively removes Ca from the cytoplasm into the lumina of the longitudinal tubules. This causes $[Ca]_i$ to fall into the range of $10^{-7}M$ (with contribution of Na-Ca exchange and the possible contribution of the SL Ca pump), and complete relaxation occurs.

The release of Ca is believed to occur from the junctional SR, which is closely apposed to the SL (see "Ultrastructure" section). Fabiato[8] has defined this release process and documented the mechanism of Ca-induced release of Ca. An amount of Ca not sufficient to activate the myofilaments directly is capable of inducing a secondary release of Ca from the SR. The release is sensitive to the rate of change of free Ca at the SR surface and to the extent of SR Ca loading. It is visualized that the initial rapid influx of Ca through the SL channel activates Ca release. Subsequent slower entry would then contribute to reloading in addition to sequestration of Ca from the longitudinal elements. The next action potential with opening of the Ca channel would, again, induce the next cycle. A free $[Ca]_i$ of about 5.5 × $10^{-7}M$ in the rat ventricle is the optimal concentration for triggering Ca release; $[Ca]_i$ values that are capable of direct activation of the myofilaments actually inhibit the Ca-induced release process.

Ventricles of different species demonstrate different dependency on Ca from the SR as compared with Ca derived directly through the trans-SL route.[10, 40] The relative dependency is demonstrated with the use of ryanodine, a drug that removes the contribution to contraction of Ca from the SR. Application of ryanodine to rat ventricle produces a decrease in force to 15% to 20% of control level. By contrast, the ryanodine response of rabbit ventricle leaves contractile force at 80% to 85% of control. Other evidence also supports the concept that the rabbit is much more dependent for direct activation on trans-SL−derived Ca than is the rat. There are no definitive data as to dependency of the human ventricle on directly activating vs. Ca-induced release of Ca for contraction, but an early study[41] would indicate the human is closer to the rabbit than to the rat. The rat ventricle is, in many respects, more similar to skeletal muscle than are the ventricles of many other mammalian species. The rat ventricle has a very rapid twitch response and a short action potential with little plateau. Such tissue seems to require an intracellular Ca release site for adequate and rapid excitation-contraction (EC) coupling. I believe it fair to state that maintenance and control of EC coupling in mammalian heart requires variable amounts of directly activating and Ca-induced release of Ca, depending on the species.

Mitochondria

The mitochondria occupy a large volume (see "Ultrastructure" section) within the cell and have an inner membrane area 16- and 40-fold greater than the membrane areas of SR and SL, respectively.[42] Though the mitochondria do not contribute to the beat-to-beat movements of Ca in the cell, they do serve as a significant Ca buffer.

Calcium uptake by the mitochondria is carrier mediated. The carrier is driven in its movement by a large inside negative potential across the inner mitochondrial membrane. The potential can be derived from an ATP-dependent pumping of protons (H^+) out of the mitochondria or by a respiration-dependent ejection of protons. The latter involves energy released by electrons moving down the respiratory chain, and this energy is conserved by the ejection of protons.[43] This ejection establishes a negative potential across the inner mitochondrial membrane, and this potential can be utilized for Ca uptake. The protonmotive force can also be converted to ATP production by an inner-membrane ATPase as protons move back into the mitochondria. This ATP can then be used to generate the negative membrane potential, which is the form of energy used to support Ca uptake. Oligomycin is an inhibitor of mitochondrial ATPase. It therefore inhibits ATP-dependent Ca uptake but permits the respiration-dependent uptake to proceed. Respiratory inhibitors, on the other hand, such as antimycin A, block the respiratory-dependent uptake, but ATP-dependent uptake may continue.

The K_m for Ca uptake is critically dependent on the Mg concentration. At physiologic $[Mg]_i$ (1 to 3 mM), the K_m is in the area of 70 μM.[44] Since, under normal physiologic conditions, $[Ca]_i$ is between 0.1 and 5 μM during the cardiac cycle, it is clear why the mitochondria play no role in the beat-to-beat control of Ca movement. But, as stated previously, as $[Ca]_i$ increases into a pathologic range, the mitochondria's huge capacity plays a role in buffering intracellular Ca. As discussed above, mitochondria generate energy through the respiratory electron-transport chain and the development of a protonmotive force. At normal $[Ca]_i$, the organelles use this force to generate ATP from ADP. This is the major responsibility of the mitochondria. However, as $[Ca]_i$ rises under pathologic conditions, the Ca uptake system is activated and energy begins to be shunted from ATP production to Ca uptake. Therefore, a condition in which the cell is subjected to a high Ca uptake, such as reperfusion after ischemia, may activate mitochondrial Ca uptake and, at the same time, produce a reduction in ATP production by the mitochondria.

The efflux of Ca from the mitochondria could be regulated by changes of the membrane potential. This would, however, be disadvantageous to the cell since so much of its metabolism is based on the maintenance of this potential. The major pathway for efflux is a carrier similar to the one described for the SL—an Na-Ca exchanger that operates to produce an Na-induced Ca release.[45] Its K_m is about 8mM of Na, which is close to the physiologic level in the cell. The system is electrogenic, thus indicating transport of more than 2 Na ions for each Ca.[46] If the mitochondria are heavily loaded with Ca, a rise in intracellular Na will increase Ca efflux to the cytosol, which would add to the increased Ca uptake via the SL Na-Ca exchanger. Therefore, cytosolic Ca would be increased from an intracellular source (mitochondria) and an extracellular source (trans-SL).

Myofilaments

The systems discussed up to this point function largely to control the Ca concentration at the myofilaments, which are the force-generating sites in the cell. Four proteins are critically involved in the response to Ca ion: myosin, actin, tropomyosin, and troponin.

Tropomyosin lies in the groove formed by the helical configuration of the strands of actin. Also attached at intervals on the actin is the three-component troponin molecule.[47] Troponin C (TNC) is the component that binds Ca, troponin I (TNI) is inhibitory, and troponin T (TNT) interacts with tropomyosin. As $[Ca]_i$ increases above 10^{-7}M, Ca binding to TNC increases. As this occurs, there is a steric effect on TNI and TNT that is believed to produce a shift of the tropomyosin molecule in the actin groove such that it "moves out of the way" and permits attachment of the myosin head to the actin. It is the troponin molecule that is responsible for the Ca sensitivity of the myofilaments. More specifically, it is the TNC component that is the end point of contractile control by Ca in the cell. It should be noted that the effect of Ca binding to TNC is to remove an inhibition to contraction, i.e., removal of the tropomyosin blockage of cross-bridge formation between actin and myosin. The removal of inhibition is graded between about 10^{-7}M and 5×10^{-6}M of $[Ca]_i$. The troponin-tropomyosin system is responsible for the Ca sensitivity of the myofilaments. Actin and myosin will remain coupled and force will be maintained until Ca is removed from TNC. If Ca removal is not complete during diastole, tension will persist and the muscle will be in a degree of contracture. Contracture, which depends on the level of $[Ca]_i$, should not be confused with rigor. Rigor can occur in the absence of Ca and refers to the state in which there is insufficient ATP to permit breakage of cross-bridges and relaxation. Both Ca-dependent contracture and ATP-deficient rigor will, of course, be manifest as an increase in diastolic tension.

Summary of Ca Movement

Figure 3 is a schematic representation of a ventricular action potential with a simultaneous trace of tension in the ventricular wall. The numbers refer to points on the action potential, the letters to phases of wall tension.

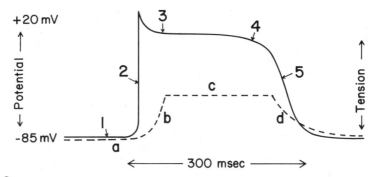

FIG 3.
Ventricular action potential as related to force development of the ventricle. See text for description of related ionic conductances and fluxes. The *numbers* refer to points or phases of the action potential, the *letters* to phases of wall force.

Point 1 is during diastole, preexcitation. The $\bar{g}_{Ca}$ is low and resting Ca flux is low; $[Ca]_i$ is under $10^{-7}M$. The SL Ca pump may be pumping small amounts of Ca out of the cell. The Na-Ca exchanger is operating to produce net movement of Na inward and Ca outward. At the myofilaments, tropomyosin inhibits actin-myosin interaction. There is no actively developed tension in the ventricular wall *(a)*.

Point 2 is the rapid phase of depolarization. The $\bar{g}_{Ca}$ increases as the membrane depolarizes to -30 to -40 mV. Calcium influx rapidly increases and $[Ca]_i$ begins to rise. The Na-Ca exchanger is still operating to produce net inward Na and net outward Ca movement, and V_E (reversal potential) for the exchanger becomes more positive. The influx of Ca through the slow channels causes a net gain of intracellular Ca. Calcium proceeds directly to the myofilaments and also induces release from the SR. Calcium binds to TNC of troponin in increasing amounts as $[Ca]_i$ rises above $10^{-7}M$ and wall tension begins to rise in the isovolumic phase *(b)* of contraction.

Point 3 to 4 is the plateau phase of depolarization. The $\bar{g}_{Ca}$ is still high but declining as channel openings become less frequent. Calcium-induced Ca release slows and Ca uptake by the SR becomes activated. Early in this period, Ca binding to TNC is maximal, and inhibition of the tropomyosin block to actin-myosin cross-bridge formation reaches a peak. This coincides with the most rapid rate of isovolumic force development during phase *b*. As wall tension results in a level of intraventricular pressure to match the diastolic pressure in pulmonary artery or aorta, the isotonic or ejection phase *(c)* begins. This phase occurs largely coincident with the action potential plateau.

Point 5 is repolarization. The $\bar{g}_{Ca}$ decreases to the resting level as channels close. Calcium influx returns to the resting level. The Na-Ca exchanger increases net outward Ca movement, and the SR is actively sequestering Ca. The decrease in Ca influx, the removal of Ca from the cell via the Na-Ca exchanger, and the sequestration by the SR results in $[Ca]_i$ falling to $10^{-7}M$ or less. Calcium leaves TNC, and tropomyosin swings back to prevent cross-bridge formation. The ventricular wall relaxes *(d)*, and the cardiac cycle is completed.

Pathology

The previous sections have focused on the movements of Ca under physiologic conditions. This final section will summarize, briefly, Ca movements under the influence of ischemia and reperfusion. It is generally agreed that many of the problems secondary to ischemia are attributable to its effects on the handling of Ca by the cell.

Within a few seconds of the onset of ischemia, there is a decline in the rate of relaxation followed by a fall in active force development.[48] The slowing of relaxation indicates that the rate of SR Ca pumping may be the most vulnerable of the cell's activities. This occurs long before a significant decrease of cellular ATP level and cannot, therefore, be easily related to a lack of energy supply unless there is a compartmentalization of an energy pool for the SR. There is no evidence for this. There is, however, evidence that the free energy change for ATP hydrolysis[49] may decline very rapidly. This represents the maximum work available from ATP hydrolysis and is equal to $-\Delta G° + RT \ln (ATP/ADP[P_i])$, where $\Delta G°$ is standard free energy change and P_i is inorganic phosphate. Though with ischemia ATP declines slowly, there is a rapid increase in ADP and $[P_i]$ levels in the cytoplasm. The free energy change required for Ca pumping by the SR is 52 kilojoules/mole, which is the highest among the cardiac ion-pumping systems (Na pump, SR Ca pump, SL Ca pump). From the formula for free energy change (above), it can be seen that a rise in the denominator may cause the free energy to fall below the level required for maintenance of SR Ca pumping before there is significant decline in ATP. This mechanism has been proposed by Kammermeier et al.[50] and would be consistent with the observed slowing of relaxation. It might even explain the decrease in active force development if impaired SR sequestration led to subsequent decrease in Ca-induced Ca release.

The role of $\Delta G°$ in reduction of active force is, however, called into question by the recent study of Kentish,[51] in which P_i was found to produce a large inhibition of Ca sensitivity of the cardiac myofibrils. It was noted that an increase of $[P_i]$ from 2 to 20 mM produced an 80% decline in force development. More significantly, it was found that if the denominator $(ADP[P_i])$ in the $\Delta G°$ equation were kept constant, with different values of ATP and P_i, there was little effect on force when ADP was increased but a major effect with increased P_i. There is evidence that P_i decreases the number of force-generating cross-bridges between actin and myosin in the presence of a fixed amount of Ca, i.e., contractile protein sensitivity is decreased. It seems possible that with ischemia, the rapid decrease in rate of relaxation is related to the inability of the SR to sustain its rate of Ca uptake, and the decrease in active force production is related to a decline in contractile protein Ca sensitivity secondary to increased $[P_i]$.

As ischemia is prolonged for up to an hour, there is little evidence that the intracellular distribution of ions, including Ca, changes significantly.[52] Diastolic tension rises, but this is due to ATP-deficient rigor and not Ca-dependent contracture. The maintenance of near-normal intracellular ion distribution indicates that SL integrity is maintained for a considerable period of ischemia. It should be noted, however, that in the presence of total ischemia the cell is only exposed to the amount of Ca within the immediate interstitial space, which is in the range of 400 μmole/kg wet weight. This is a relatively low "Ca load," which might be handled by the cell even if the SL were to become somewhat "leaky" during the ischemic period.

The situation changes dramatically on reperfusion after an hour of ischemia. Two groups of cells can be identified.[52] One group retains essentially normal ionic distribution and would seem to remain viable, whereas another population demonstrates an intracellular ionic distribution little different from that of the extracellular medium. These cells show disrupted SL with peeling of the glycocalyx and evidence of high Ca loading with Ca-apatite precipitation in the mitochondria. There is marked contracture of the myofilaments. These characteristics are typical of cell death. It seems likely that an important factor in the determination of which group, living or dead, a cell will join on reperfusion is whether or not SL integrity is maintained.

The sequence of events leading to disruption of the SL remains controversial at this time, but there is evidence for the following scheme.[53, 54] During prolonged ischemia there is a progressive decline in ATP, with ATP $\rightarrow$ AMP $\rightarrow$ adenosine $\rightarrow$ inosine $\rightarrow$ hypoxanthine $\rightarrow$ xanthine. In the presence of xanthine dehydrogenase and oxidized nicotinamide adenine dinucleotide (NAD^+), the following reaction occurs: $-$ xanthine $+ H_2O + NAD^+ \xrightarrow{\text{xanthine dehydrogenase}}$ uric acid $+$ reduced NAD (NADH) $+ H^+$. The products are innocuous and do not result in membrane damage. However, if on reperfusion the SL is leaky, an elevation of cytosolic Ca occurs. This results in activation of a protease that converts the xanthine dehydrogenase to xanthine oxidase. Under these conditions and with re-supply of oxygen, the reaction is: xanthine $+ H_2O + O_2 \xrightarrow{\text{xanthine oxidase}}$ uric acid $+ 2O_2^- + 2H^+$. The O_2^- is the superoxide radical, a molecule with an odd number of electrons, which renders it very reactive chemically. This radical can react with lipid hydroperoxides to form destructive alkoxy radicals in the SL or the free radicals can be converted to hydrogen peroxide if an adequate amount of superoxide dismutase (SOD) is present: $2O_2^- + 2H^+ \xrightarrow{\text{SOD}} H_2O_2 + O_2$. If there is now sufficient catalase present, the H_2O_2 is converted: $2H_2O_2 \xrightarrow{\text{catalase}} O_2 + 2H_2O$. If sufficient catalase is not present, then H_2O_2 in the presence of ferrous iron produces the very destructive hydroxyl radical ($^{\cdot}OH$): $Fe^{2+} + H_2O_2 \rightarrow Fe^{3+} + {^{\cdot}OH} + OH^-$. The ($^{\cdot}OH$) radical is potent in the production of lipid peroxides in the membrane. This increases SL fluidity, leading to increased permeability and loss of integrity. This promotes further increase in cytosolic Ca, leading to further production of xanthine oxidase as well as to activation of other enzymes, such as phospholipase A_2, which will add to phospholipid hydrolysis, with additional loss of SL integrity. A vicious cycle is established. The initial leak of Ca activates enzymes, leading to further membrane destruction, which leads to additional Ca leakage.

From the scheme presented it is apparent that, upon reperfusion, SL damage can be avoided in either of two ways: (1) the ischemic period does not produce sufficient membrane damage to permit enough Ca leakage to produce the initial xanthine oxidase formation; (2) even though free radicals are produced, there is adequate SOD and catalase present to "scavenge" them and prevent their destructive interaction with the membrane lipid. There are a number of studies indicating that the administration of free radical scavengers produces significant amelioration of reperfusion injury.[55, 56]

Conclusion

Whereas voluntary skeletal muscle can modulate its contractile force by recruitment of more or fewer motor units, cardiac muscle has no such mechanism. It is an "all or none" muscle. Either all cells contract or none contract. This means that force must be modulated within each individual cell. This is done through the Frank-Starling length-tension relationship for response to preload changes. Virtually all other responses involve control of the concentration of Ca at the sarcomeric myofilaments. This is accomplished in the mammalian heart through interaction of processes at the SL and SR. The SL phenomena include Ca binding, flux through a specific channel and via the Na-Ca exchanger, and operation of an SL Ca pump. The SR phenomena include Ca pumping and Ca-induced Ca release. Force development can be modified by a change in any one or any combination of these processes.

The response to myocardial ischemia, and whether or not the injury sustained will be reversible on reperfusion, is critically dependent on maintenance of SL integrity, particularly with respect to its Ca permeability. High Ca permeability can lead to the establishment of a vicious cycle of Ca entry leading to SL damage, then increased Ca entry, further SL damage, further Ca entry, further SL damage, and finally cell death.

References

1. Allen DG, Kentish JC: The cellular basis of the length-tension relation in cardiac muscle. *J Mol Cell Cardiol* 1985; 17:821–840.
2. Langer GA, Frank JS, Philipson KD: Ultrastructure and calcium exchange of the sarcolemma, sarcoplasmic reticulum and mitochondria of the myocardium. *Pharmacol Ther* 1982; 16:331–376.
3. Langer GA, Frank JS, Nudd LM, et al: Sialic acid: Effect of removal on calcium exchangeability of cultured heart cells. *Science* 1976; 193:1013–1015.
4. Jennings RB, Ganote CE, Reimer KA: Ischemic tissue injury. *Am J Pathol* 1975; 81:179–198.
5. Singer SL, Nicolson GL: The fluid mosaic model of the structure of cell membranes. *Science* 1972; 175:720–731.
6. Cooper DL, Goodenough DA, Makowski L, et al: Gap junction structures: I. Correlated electron microscopy and x-ray diffraction. *J Cell Biol* 1977; 74:605–645.
7. Endo M, Tanaka M, Ogawa Y: Calcium-induced release of calcium from the sarcoplasmic reticulum of skeletal muscle fibers. *Nature* 1970; 228:34–36.
8. Fabiato A: Calcium-induced release of calcium from cardiac sarcoplasmic reticulum. *Am J Physiol* 1983; 245:C1–C14.
9. Armstrong CM, Bezanilla FM, Horawicz P: Twitches in the presence of ethylene glycol bis (β-aminoethylether)-N-N'tetraacetic acid. *Biochim Biophys Acta* 1972; 267:605–608.
10. Rich TL, Langer GA, Klassen MG: Two components of coupling calcium in the single ventricular cell of rabbits and rats. *Am J Physiol,* 1988; 254: H937–H946.

11. Page E, McCallister P: Quantitative electron-microscopic description of heart muscle cells: Application to normal, hypertrophied and thyroxin-stimulated hearts. *Am J Cardiol* 1973; 31:172–181.
12. Bers DM, Langer GA: Upcoupling cation effects on cardiac contractility and sarcolemmal Ca^{2+} binding. *Am J Physiol* 1979; 237:H332–H341.
13. Langer GA: Role of sarcolemmal-bound Ca in regulation of myocardial contractile force. *J Am Coll Cardiol* 1986; 8:65A–68A.
14. Fintel M, Langer GA, Rohloff JC, et al: Contribution of myocardial diffuse double layer calcium to contractile function. *Am J Physiol* 1985; 249:H989–H994.
15. McLaughlin A, Eng W, Vaio G, et al: Dimethonium, a divalent cation that exerts only a screening effect on the electrostatic potential adjacent to negatively charged phospholipid bilayer membranes. *J Membr Biol* 1983; 76:183–193.
16. Noma A, Misawa H: Membrane currents in the rabbit sinoatrial node cell as studied by the double microelectrode method. *Pflugers Arch* 1976; 364:45–52.
17. Kokubun A, Nishimura M, Noma A, et al: Membrane currents in the rabbit atrioventricular node cell. *Pflugers Arch* 1982; 393:15–22.
18. Schramm M, Thomas G, Towart R, et al: Novel dihydropyridines with positive inotropic action through activation of Ca^{2+} channels. *Nature* 1983; 303:535–537.
19. Kuo JF, Greengard P: Cyclic-nucleotide dependent protein kinases: IV. Widespread occurrence of adenosine 3′,5′monophosphate-dependent protein kinase in various tissues and phyla of the animal kingdom. *Proc Natl Acad Sci USA* 1969; 64:1349–1355.
20. Greengard P: Phosphorylated proteins as physiological effectors. *Science* 1978; 199:146–152.
21. Tsien R: Cyclic AMP and contractile activity in heart, in Greengard P, Robinson GA (eds): *Advances in Nucleotide Research*. New York, Raven Press, 1977, pp 363–420.
22. Ten Eick R, Nawrath H, McDonald T, et al: On the mechanism of the negative inotropic effect of acetylcholine. *Pflugers Arch* 1976; 361:207–213.
23. George WJ, Wilkersen RD, Kadowitz PJ: Influence of acetylcholine on contractile force and cyclic nucleotide levels in isolated perfused heart. *J Pharmacol Exp Ther* 1973; 184:228–235.
24. Nawrath H: Does cyclic GMP mediate the negative inotropic effect of acetylcholine in the heart? *Nature* 1977; 267:72–74.
25. Lüttgau HC, Niedergerke R: The antagonism between Ca and Na ions on the frog's heart. *J Physiol* 1958; 143:486–505.
26. Repke K: Über den biochemischen Wirkingsmodus von Digitalis. *Klin Wochenschr* 1964; 42:157–165.
27. Langer GA: Kinetic studies of calcium distribution in ventricular muscle of the dog. *Circ Res* 1964; 15:393–405.
28. Reuter H, Seitz N: The dependence of calcium efflux from cardiac muscle on temperature and external ion composition. *J Physiol* 1968; 195:451–470.
29. Baker PF, Blaustein MP, Hodgkin AL, et al: The influence of calcium on sodium efflux in squid axons. *J Physiol* 1969; 200:431–458.
30. Benninger C, Einwachter HM, Haas HG, et al: Calcium-sodium antagonism on the frog's heart: A voltage clamp study. *J Physiol* 1976; 259:617–645.
31. Reeves JP, Hale CC: The stoichiometry of the cardiac sodium-calcium exchange system. *J Biol Chem* 1984; 259:7732–7739.

32. Cohn CJ, Fozzard HA, Sheu SS: Increase in intracellular sodium ion activity during stimulation in mammalian cardiac muscle. Circ Res 1982; 50:651–662.

33. Langer GA: Ion fluxes in cardiac excitation and contraction and their relation to myocardial contractility. Physiol Rev 1968; 48:708–757.

34. Withering W: An account of the foxglove and some of its medical uses with practical remarks on dropsy and other diseases. London, GGJ & J Robinson, 1785. Reprinted in Williams FA, Keys TE (eds): Cardiac Classics. St Louis, CV Mosby Co, 1941; pp 227–252.

35. Langer GA: The intrinsic control of myocardial contraction: Ionic factors. N Engl J Med 1971; 285:1065–1071.

36. Lee CO, Kang DH, Sokol JH, et al: Relation between intracellular Na ion activity and tension in sheep cardiac Purkinje fibers exposed to dihydro-ouabain. Biophys J 1980; 29:315–330.

37. Caroni P, Carafoli E: An ATP dependent Ca-pumping system in the dog heart sarcolemma. Nature 1980; 283:765–767.

38. Entman ML, Levey GS, Epstein SE: Mechanism of action of epinephrine and glucagon on the canine heart. Circ Res 1969; 25:429–438.

39. Tada M, Kirchberger MA, Katz AM: Phosphorylation of a 22,000-dalton component of the cardiac sarcoplasmic reticulum by adenosine 3'5'monophosphate-dependent protein kinase. J Biol Chem 1975; 250:2640–2647.

40. Bers DM: Ca influx and sarcoplasmic reticulum Ca release in cardiac muscle activation during postrest recovery. Am J Physiol 1985; 248:H366–H381.

41. Fabiato A, Fabiato F: Calcium-induced release of calcium from the sarcoplasmic reticulum of skinned cells from adult human, dog, cat, rabbit, rat and frog hearts and from fetal and new-born rat ventricles. Ann NY Acad Sci 1978; 307:491–522.

42. Page E: Quantitative ultrastructural analysis in cardiac membrane physiology. Am J Physiol 1978; 235:C147–C158.

43. Mitchell P: Keilin's respiratory chain concept and its chemiosmotic consequences. Science 1979; 206:1148–1159.

44. Scarpa A: Transport across mitochondrial membranes, in Grelisch G, Tostesen DC, Ussing HH (eds): Membrane Transport Biology. New York, Springer-Verlag New York, 1979, pp 263–355.

45. Carafoli E, Trozzo R, Lugli G, et al: The release of calcium from heart mitochondria by sodium. J Mol Cell Cardiol 1974; 6:361–371.

46. Crompton M, Kunzi M, Carafoli E: The calcium-induced and sodium-induced effluxes of calcium from heart mitochondria. Eur J Biochem 1977; 79:549–558.

47. Ebashi S: Regulatory mechanism of muscle contraction with special reference to the Ca-troponin-tropomyosin system. Essays Biochem 1974; 10:1–36.

48. Shine KI, Douglas AM, Ricchiuti NV: Ischemia in isolated interventricular septa: Mechanical events. Am J Physiol 1976; 231:1225–1232.

49. Gibbs C: The cytoplasmic phosphorylation potential: Its possible role in the control of myocardial respiration and cardiac contractility. J Mol Cell Cardiol 1985; 17:727–731.

50. Kammermeier H, Schmidt P, Jungling E: Free energy change of ATP hydrolysis: A causal factor of early hypoxic failure of the myocardium. J Mol Cell Cardiol 1982; 14:267–277.

51. Kentish JC: The effects of inorganic phosphate and creatine phosphate on force production in skinned muscles from rat ventricle. J Physiol 1986; 370:585–604.

52. Walsh L, Tormey JM: Subcellular electrolyte shifts during in vitro myocardial ischemia and reperfusion. *Am J Physiol,* 1988; 255:H917–H928..
53. McCord JM: Oxygen-derived free radicals in postischemic tissue injury. *N Engl J Med* 1985; 312:159–163.
54. Thompson JA, Hess ML: The oxygen free radical system: A fundamental mechanism in the production of myocardial necrosis. *Prog Cardiovasc Dis* 1986; 28:449–462.
55. Jolly SR, Kane WJ, Bailie MB, et al: Canine myocardial reperfusion on injury: Its reduction by the combined administration of superoxide dismutase and catalase. *Circ Res* 1984; 54:277–285.
56. Przyklenk K, Kloner RA: Superoxide dismutase plus catalase improve contractile function in the canine model of the "stunned myocardium." *Circ Res* 1986; 73:148–156.

Special Considerations in Mitral Valve and Coronary Artery Disease

Robert B. Karp, M.D.

Professor of Surgery, Chief of Cardiac Surgery, University of Chicago, Chicago, Illinois

This chapter deals with surgery for mitral valve dysfunction associated with coronary artery disease. It particularly emphasizes mitral valve regurgitation resulting from myocardial ischemic injury. Certainly, indications for and results of surgery vary in this combination of conditions. Controversy exists in some areas. However, I shall put forth seven propositions relating to the combination of mitral valve disease and coronary artery disease. I shall add supporting and also controversial information from the literature and then discuss further results and long-term outcomes. Finally, I shall propose a plan of management.

Seven Propositions

Proposition 1

The degree of mitral regurgitation, when associated with coronary artery disease, may be difficult to define and quantitate. Five objective findings that may be useful in attempting to assess the degree of mitral regurgitation are the murmur, the chest roentgenogram, the echo Doppler findings, results of angiocardiography and left ventriculography, and findings at operation.

In severe mitral regurgitation of an acute nature, the murmur tends to decrease in intensity or be absent in late systole. Occasionally, there is a crescendo-decrescendo configuration. Varieties of papillary muscle dysfunction may present as a midsystolic or late systolic or even early systolic murmur.[1] The murmurs may be associated with atrial fourth sounds and left ventricular third sounds or gallops. Heikkila[2] reports that 50% of patients during or recovering from myocardial infarction at one time or another present a systolic murmur of mitral regurgitation. The murmur then can be variable and evanescent and, like mitral incompetence itself, come and go with variations of ischemia. The murmur depends also on the presence or absence of silent ischemia. It may occur only during angina. It may vary with the degree of hydration of the patient and may be associated with and result from ST-T wave changes.

Adv Card Surg 1:77–92, 1990

The chest roentgenogram is useful to corroborate hemodynamic findings. However, isolated left ventricular dysfunction, whether it be systolic or diastolic, may cause pulmonary venous engorgement and roentgenographic findings of pulmonary venous hypertension. Usually, in ischemic mitral regurgitation, the left atrium is small or only mildly enlarged, and thus chamber enlargement is not a satisfactory parameter by which to judge the degree of mitral regurgitation.

Nagel and colleagues[3] have proposed angiographic criteria for mitral regurgitation graded 1, mild; 2, moderate; and 3, severe. In ischemic mitral regurgitation, the degree of regurgitation may vary with the state of hydration, the left ventricular end diastolic pressure, or the position of the left ventricular catheter, and also be modified by frequent premature ventricular contractions. The degree of ischemia at the time of angiography, of course, is a major factor that must be considered when judging the degree of mitral regurgitation.

Helmcke and colleagues,[4] using color Doppler and echocardiographic techniques, found a good correlation between Doppler and angiocardiographic degree of mitral regurgitation. The sensitivity and specificity of color Doppler for detecting mitral regurgitation, were 100% in 147 patients evaluated. Additionally, the correlation between the degree of mitral regurgitation by angiography and by color Doppler was $r = .78$. In my experience, color Doppler may be used in a serial fashion to estimate the presence and severity of mitral regurgitation. However, simply one or two Doppler examinations may not give the final picture as to the severity.

Operative assessment can be done before cardiopulmonary bypass by palpation of the regurgitant jet posteriorly behind the inferior vena cava and anteriorly at the roof of the left atrium below the root of the aorta. A regurgitant bruit felt anteriorly indicates a major posterior leaflet problem, and similarly a posterior jet suggests an anterior leaflet problem. Additional information may be occasionally obtained by the pulmonary artery wedge tracing or after insertion of a small polyvinyl catheter into the left atrium. Again, however, this depends on the state of ischemia and the loading conditions of the heart at the time the estimations are made. Often, visual inspection of the mitral valve may be misleading as to the degree of mitral incompetence. Certainly, the presence of mitral incompetence may be confirmed, but the severity cannot be accurately graded.

Therefore, decision making based solely on one or two estimates may be misleading when mitral regurgitation is associated with ischemic heart disease. As noted above, I suggest serial examinations, by both auscultation and color Doppler, along with an assessment of the degree of pulmonary venous hypertension to lead one to make an accurate assessment of the severity of the mitral regurgitation.

Proposition 2

The severity of mitral regurgitation may vary. The degree of mitral regurgitation, when due to coronary artery disease and following a myocardial infarction, may wax and wane over time. As noted, this is particularly true when loading conditions are varied by treatment modalities and the degree of ischemia varies, owing to either spontaneous changes in the coronary blood flow or therapeutic manipulations. As a rule, the severity will become less as time goes on, except in the most severe cases or those cases where there are clear-cut anatomic distortions such as papillary muscle scarring or chordal rupture. An exception to the statement that mitral regurgitation in ischemic heart disease will improve over time is the situation in which there is papillary muscle rupture (as opposed to papillary muscle dysfunction). In reality, papillary muscle rupture is rupture of a portion of the head of a papillary muscle. Papillary muscle rupture is a surgical emergency. It occurs in less than 1% of myocardial infarctions and cannot be tolerated by the patient for more than 6 to 8 hours.

It can be stated, therefore, that mitral regurgitation due to coronary artery disease exhibits a tendency to clarify its severity over time. This tendency, however, can be affected by transients or new ischemia and variations in loading conditions.

Proposition 3

The cardiac status of a patient with mitral regurgitation due to coronary artery disease is very nearly equal to a cardiomyopathy. It exhibits a dim prognosis, much more severe than either isolated mitral regurgitation or mitral regurgitation associated with but not etiologically related to coronary artery disease. Thus, the outcome of mitral regurgitation due to coronary artery disease is related both to the severity of left ventricular dysfunction and to the severity of the mitral regurgitation.

For example, Balu et al.[5] examined the fate of 104 patients with mitral regurgitation and coronary artery disease. Sixty of these were thought to have mitral regurgitation on an ischemic basis. Follow-up was reported on 43 who were treated medically and 12 who were treated surgically. Follow-up was unavailable for five surgical patients, three of whom refused postoperative evaluation and two of whom died. At 18.5 months' follow-up, survival in the medical group was 57.5% compared with 90% in the surgical group. Thus, in less than 2 years, about 40% of patients with ischemic mitral regurgitation were dead (Fig 1).

Proposition 4

It is possible to repair (rather than replace) the mitral valve more frequently than has been suggested in the past. Traditionally, and even at present, angiographic and surgical assessment of the mitral valve is less than perfect to judge correctly the anatomic cause of the mitral regurgitation. This has led to two problems. The first is the establishment of the correct or best reparative procedure or procedures to produce a competent valve. Second, the desire to attain a perfectly competent valve in these poorly functioning left ventricles often leads to replacement. Replacement, so the rea-

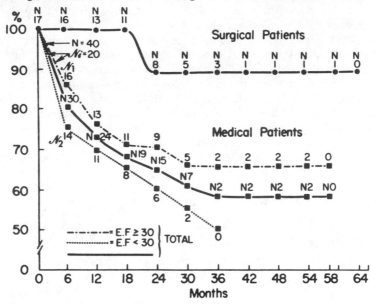

FIG 1.
The number of patients followed up for a period is plotted on the x axis and the percentage survival on the y axis. The difference in survival for the medical group is according to the EF, $n_1 \geq 30\%$ and $n_2 < 30\%$. From Balu V, Hershowitz S, Masud ARZ, et al: Mitral regurgitation in coronary artery disease. *Chest* 1982; 81:550–555. Used by permission.)

soning goes, will remove one variable in the postoperative equation for the identification of the cause and treatment of low cardiac output.

The recent trend toward mitral valve repair (in isolated mitral regurgitation) supports this new attitude to attempt repair in ischemic mitral incompetence. However, much of the data on the success of repair come from procedures done on nonischemic mitral valve disease.[6, 7]

There is, furthermore, some information that left ventricular function is preserved when repair is done compared with replacement. However, those data originate generally from operations done in patients with good left ventricular performance, i.e., ejection fractions greater than 55%.[8] Additionally, the data on repair are derived from patients with isolated mitral valve regurgitation, not due to left ventricular dysfunction secondary to ischemia.

A long-time proponent of repair in ischemic mitral regurgitation is Jerome Kay. In 1986, Kay et al.[9] reported on 141 patients who underwent either repair (101 patients) or replacement (40 patients). Repair was associated with better short- and long-term survival than was valve replacement, especially in patients with low ejection fractions (Fig 2). Strangely, operative mortality was not included in the report. It is notable, however, that 70% of patients were candidates for repair in the Kay et al. series.

Proposition 5

Only severe mitral regurgitation necessitates repair or valve replacement. Because of variation of intensity of regurgitation and the independent effects of the degree of coronary artery disease, wall motion score, ejection fraction, and remoteness of infarction (among others), it is reasonable to suggest that only the severest regurgitation necessitates repair or replacement. Pinson and colleagues[10] of Starr's group concluded such. They reported on 120 patients with ischemic mitral regurgitation and coronary artery disease. Eighty-three patients had coronary artery bypass grafting alone and 37 also had a valve operation. All patients with mild mitral regurgitation (67 patients) were treated with coronary artery bypass grafting alone as compared with 14 of 21 patients with moderate and two of 32 with severe mitral regurgitation. Operative mortalities were 4%, 10%, and 38%, respectively. Long-term survival, depicted as in Figure 3 from Starr's

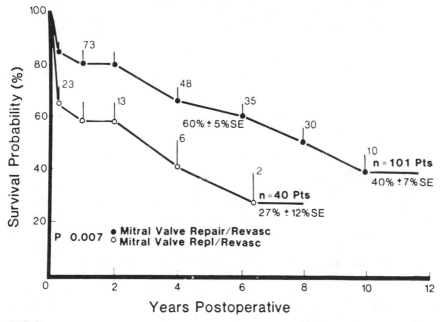

FIG 2.
Probability of survival for patients undergoing mitral repair and those receiving a mitral valve replacement, operative mortality included. *Revasc* = revascularization; *Repl* = replacement. (From Kay GL, Kay JH, Zubiate P, et al: Mitral valve repair for mitral regurgitation secondary to coronary artery disease. *Circulation* 1986; 74:188–198. Used by permission.)

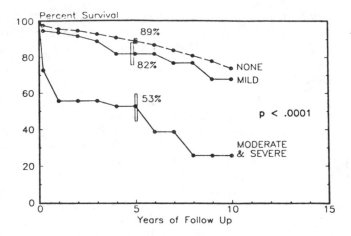

FIG 3.
Survival as a function of the severity of ischemic mitral regurgitation. Five-year cumulative proportions surviving are shown, and SEs are indicated by the bars. Survival for patients without mitral regurgitation who required coronary bypass is shown for comparison. The *P* value refers to the difference between the regurgitation groups only. (From Pinson CW, Cobanoglu A, Metzdorff MT, et al: Late surgical results for ischemic mitral regurgitation: Role of wall motion score and severity of regurgitation. *J Thorac Cardiovasc Surg* 1984; 88:663–672. Used by permission.)

group, is related to the severity of mitral regurgitation. Severe wall motion abnormalities were also a powerful determinant of survival. Pinson and colleagues suggest that severe mitral regurgitation is comparable to multiple paradoxic segmental wall dysfunction and should, therefore, be eliminated when severe.

Proposition 6

It is a fact that when mitral regurgitation is the result of coronary artery disease, the operative and long-term survival is less good than when (1) the mitral regurgitation and coronary artery disease are associated but not etiologically related, (2) only one of the two exists as the indication for operation, or (3) there is a mixed mitral lesion. Early information regarding these conclusions came from Salomon et al.[11] in a Stanford study published in 1977. Those authors identified coronary artery disease in mitral valve regurgitation as an important risk factor for operative survival. They also noted that the primary cause of mitral valve disease had a significant effect on long-term survival (Fig 4). Another study, now 10 years old, by Chaffin and Daggett[12] simply identified ungrafted coronary artery disease as a major risk factor for death after mitral valve replacement (Fig 5). Andrade et al.[13] did not specifically find ischemic etiology of mitral valve regurgitation to be a risk factor in operative survival. However, wall motion score was a powerful risk factor. If one interprets a

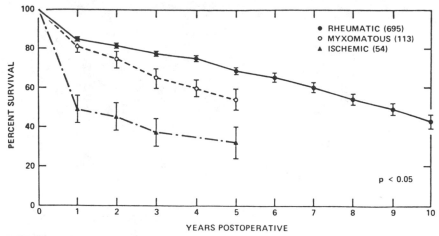

FIG 4.
Influence of the primary cause (rheumatic, myxomatous, ischemic) of mitral valve disease on postoperative actuarial survival. (From Salomon NW, Stinson EB, Griepp RB, et al: Patient-related risk factors as predictors of results following isolated mitral valve replacement. *Ann Thorac Surg* 1977; 24:519–530. Used by permission.)

high wall motion score (greater segmental wall motion abnormalities) to reflect ischemic etiology, then in the article by Andrade et al., in fact, mitral regurgitation caused by coronary artery disease had worse survival (Fig 6,A and 6,B).

Finally, at the University of Alabama, Birmingham, we found a higher operative mortality and worse long-term survival in patients with mitral valve regurgitation when the mitral regurgitation was the result of coronary artery disease. Operative mortality was 17% in ischemic mitral regurgitation, compared with 4.5% for nonischemic mitral valve disease. An impressive testament to the deleterious effect of mitral regurgitation caused by coronary artery disease was reported by Czer and associates.[15] They found a 19.8% operative mortality in patients with coronary artery bypass grafting and mitral valve regurgitation when the coronary artery disease was etiologically related to the mitral regurgitation. This compared with a 7.3% operative mortality when only an incidental relationship was present between coronary artery disease and mitral valve disease (Fig 7).

Proposition 7

To deal with mitral regurgitation in coronary artery disease, one must recognize that several factors are causal. The suspected or possible causes of mitral regurgitation in ischemic heart disease result from the following: (1) geometric (dilatation of the ventricular chamber, lengthening of the minor axis, etc); (2) papillary muscle dysfunction (scarring, lengthening, ischemia,

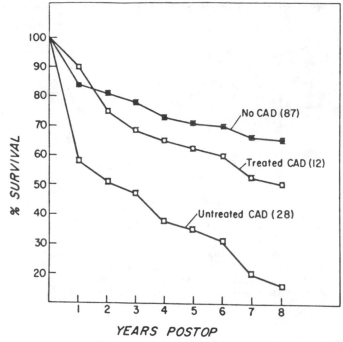

FIG 5.
Probability of survival after mitral valve replacement in patients without coronary artery disease (CAD), with CAD but no grafting, and with CAD and saphenous vein grafting. *Postop* = postoperative. (From Chaffin JS, Daggett WM: Mitral valve replacement: A 9-year follow-up of risks and survival. *Ann Thorac Surg* 1979; 27:312–319. Used by permission.)

etc); (3) anular dilatation; (4) chordal stretch or rupture (leading to prolapse [one of several types of prolapse]); (5) left ventricular dilatation (long and minor axis elongation).

Finally, the factors enumerated above help to define ischemic mitral regurgitation, as opposed to primary prolapse, myxedematous changes, rheumatic changes, or mitral regurgitation associated with but not etiologically related to coronary artery disease. Kay et al.[9] described anular dilatation as a constant finding in ischemic mitral regurgitation. However, a majority of their patients also had papillary muscle or chordal abnormalities. Czer et al.,[15] in their report, concluded that there was an ischemic etiology to mitral regurgitation in coronary artery disease if the patient had mitral regurgitation angiographically along with coronary artery abnormalities plus papillary muscle infarction or ischemia, mitral anular dilatation and left ventricular dilatation with healed infarction(s), and an otherwise normal mitral valve, or a combination of the above with sclerotic or myxomatous changes of the valve. For some—for example, myself and Andrade et al.—ischemic etiology is one of exclusion using the usual criteria for myx-

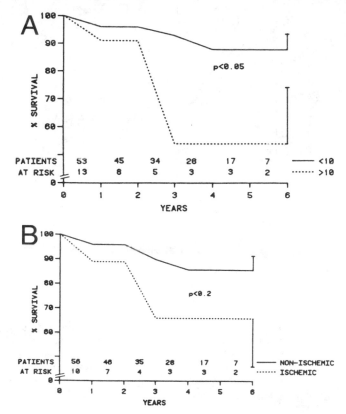

FIG 6.
A, influence of poor ventricular function (wall motion score >10) on survival with
mitral valve replacement plus coronary artery bypass grafting. A significant difference is reached between the second and third year after operation. **B,** influence of
ischemic etiology of mitral disease on survival of patients with mitral valve replacement plus coronary artery bypass grafting. Survival is shorter with ischemic mitral
disease, but the difference is not significant. (From Andrade IG, Cartier R, Panisi P,
et al: Factors influencing early and late survival in patients with combined mitral
valve replacement and myocardial revascularization and in those with isolated replacement. *Ann Thorac Surg* 1987; 44:607–613. Used by permission.)

omatous, rheumatic, and such, in the presence of a normal-appearing
valve apparatus plus previous infarctions.

Discussion

Are the foregoing seven propositions absolutely true? Probably only partially or, in some reports, absolutely not. For example, in 1982, DiSesa
and colleagues[16] reported an 18% mortality in 100 consecutive patients
having mitral valve replacement and coronary artery bypass grafting. They

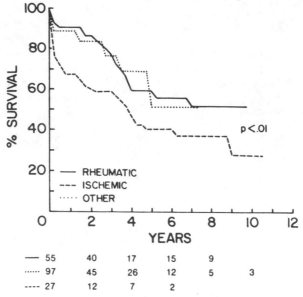

FIG 7.
Survival after combined valve replacement and revascularization, stratified by the etiology of the mitral valve disease. The 8-year survival rate in the patients with ischemic disease was 37% ± 6% compared with 52% ± 9% in patients with rheumatic or other etiologies of mitral valve disease. (From Czer LSC, Gray RJ, DeRobertis MA, et al: Mitral valve replacement: Impact of coronary artery disease and determinants of prognosis after revascularization. *Circulation* 1984; 70:1198–1207. Used by permission.)

compared this with a 23.7% mortality in a 15-institution coronary artery surgery study (CASS) report. This CASS study covered 6,630 patients, 38 of whom had mitral valve surgery. In DiSesa's experience, pulmonary vascular resistance, cardiac index, and ejection fraction were highly significant variables relating to survival. The strongest risks were New York Heart Association functional class and emergency operation. However, coronary heart disease vs. rheumatic etiology and regurgitation vs. stenosis were not predictors of operative mortality. Neither was mitral regurgitation due to coronary artery disease vs. that due to rheumatic fever, a significant determinant of mortality (Table 1).

In an accompanying editorial, we presented data that coronary artery disease certainly was a significant risk factor when the mitral valve regurgitation was etiologically related to ischemia.[14] The mortality in that group of 96 patients was 17% when there was an ischemic etiology and 9% when there was only an incidental relationship.

There may be a middle ground, inasmuch as patients with coronary artery disease more frequently present in an unstable condition and with segmental wall dysfunction. They thus fit into DiSesa's emergency or class IV group and thus have a high mortality.

TABLE 1.
Relationship Between Variables of Heart Disease and
Operative Mortality for Combined Mitral Valve
Replacement and Coronary Revascularization*†

Variable	No. of Patients	No. of Deaths	Mortality, %
Coronary artery disease	55	10	18.2
Rheumatic heart disease	45	8	17.8
Functional class‡			
III	36	0	0
IV	64	18	28.1
Mitral regurgitation	76	16	21.1
Mitral stenosis	24	2	8.3
Mitral regurgitation			
Due to coronary artery disease	55	10	18.2
Due to rheumatic heart disease	21	6	28.6

*From DiSesa VJ, Cohn LH, Collins JJ, et al: *Ann Thorac Surg* 1982; 34:482–489. Used by permission.
†In 100 patients.
‡Based on New York Heart Association criteria; class III vs. class IV, $P < .01$.

On the other hand, the concept of coronary artery disease as an etiology leading to a higher mortality is supported in reports by Connolly et al.,[17] Kay et al.[18] from Oregon, Pinson et al.,[10] Andrade et al.,[13] and Magovern et al.[19] Czer and associates[15] from Los Angeles found that coronary artery disease, etiologically related to ischemic mitral regurgitation, identified a high-risk group of patients with a 30-day mortality of 19.6%. Incidental coronary artery disease associated with mitral valve disease, on the other hand, resulted in 7.3% mortality ($P < .03$).

Along with coronary artery disease etiology, wall motion score (and its related ejection fraction, left ventricular end diastolic pressure, low grade index, and elevated pulmonary artery pressure), priority of operation, and age are usually found to be incremental risks for early hospital death after operations on the mitral valve in the presence of ischemic heart disease. Czer et al.,[15] Salomon et al.[11] and Chaffin and Daggett[12] have, in addition, clearly demonstrated that complete (or nearly complete) revascularization in that setting is superior to leaving coronary artery disease unbypassed. Long-term survival is also clearly and similarly influenced by coronary artery bypass grafting. Czer et al.[15] present their data for their total patients (Fig 8,A) and for matched cohorts of patients (Fig 8,B). In either analysis, leaving coronary artery disease unbypassed increases mortality. Thus, operative survival is less in coronary artery disease etiologically re-

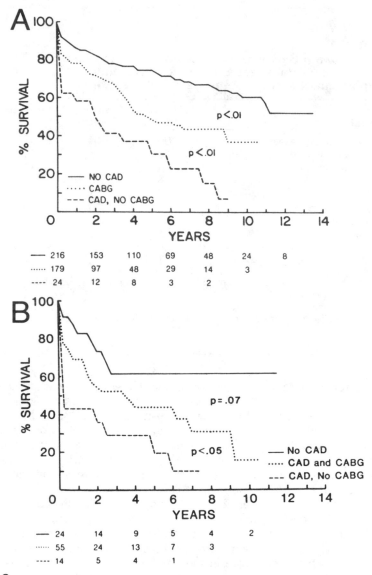

FIG 8.
A, survival after valve replacement in three cohorts of patients, stratified by presence or absence of coronary artery disease (CAD) and coronary artery bypass grafting (CABG). The 5- and 8-year survival rates and SEs were 75% ± 3% and 68% ± 4% in patients with no CAD; 49% ± 5% and 44% ± 5% in patients with bypassed CAD; and 31% ± 10% and 15% ± 9% in patients with unbypassed CAD. **B,** the cohorts have been matched in age, sex ratio, preoperative ejection fraction, and valve lesion. (From Czer LSC, Gray RJ, DeRobertis MA, et al: Mitral valve replacement: Impact of coronary artery disease and determinants of prognosis after revascularization. *Circulation* 1984; 70:1198–1207. Used by permission.)

lated to mitral regurgitation and long-term survival is probably also negatively affected, as in ischemic cardiomyopathies.

What is an ischemic mitral valve lesion? Kay et al.[9] stress the fact that ischemic mitral regurgitation is uniformly characterized by anular dilatation. Their operative technique is based on that fact. In addition, they offer the criteria in Table 2. Kay et al. give no precise figure for operative mortality but, among 101 patients with repair and 40 patients with replacement, the 6-year survival is 60% and 27%, respectively. Kay and coworkers favor a repair that shortens the posterior anulus about 70% and includes repair of torn chordae and papillary muscles. In patients with ejection fraction greater than 40%, repair has resulted in a 6-year survival of 86%, whereas replacement has generated a 56% 6-year survival. Of interest, Kay's group recommends two distinct periods of cardioplegic myocardial arrest: revascularization is done first, followed by reperfusion, then reapplication of cardioplegia, and then mitral surgery.

What then is the best plan for a patient with mitral regurgitation and coronary artery disease? In my opinion, emergency operation is indicated only in papillary muscle rupture. Mitral valve replacement is necessary, and coronary artery bypass grafting optimizes the patient's chance of functional recovery. Tepe and Edmunds[20] report five of 11 patients surviving operation.

In all other situations, stabilizing and temporizing are the watchwords. Intra-aortic balloon pumping is frequently appropriate. Often the mitral regurgitation will wax and wane and more than occasionally diminish substantially. After infarction, early coronary arteriography is performed with left ventricular angiography. The mitral regurgitation is assessed serially by auscultation and by color Doppler echocardiography.

I believe a temporizing approach will allow some patients to improve their ultimate chance of surviving operation. However, others will need urgent intervention.

It is appropriate to adhere to the admonition of Starr's group[10]: approach the mitral valve only in moderately severe or severe regurgitation. In my experience, when severe mitral regurgitation exists, about three fifths

---

TABLE 2.
Criteria for Determining That Mitral Regurgitation is Secondary to Coronary Artery Disease*

Evidence of myocardial infarction antedating the murmur of mitral regurgitation
No evidence of any connective tissue disorder
Intraoperative evidence of papillary muscle infarction or ischemic changes
Lack of intraoperative findings of mitral valve prolapse, commissural fusion, or
  other stigmata of inflammatory valve disease

*From Kay GL, Kay JH, Zubiate P, et al: Circulation 1986; 74:188–198. Used by permission.

of those patients receive mitral valve replacement, usually a xenograft. The remaining 40% are candidates for valve repair (see above 70% in the Kay et al. series). In contrast to mitral regurgitation of nonischemic etiology, a Carpentier ring anuloplasty is not used. Instead, a bicommissural anuloplasty is done. We insert a double-armed 2-0 felt buttressed polypropylene stitch anterior to each commissure and move centrally and posteriorly to shorten the posterior two thirds of the mitral ring 50% to 70%. The suture bites are similar to the deVega technique, and the result is similar to that with the "asymmetric anuloplasty" of Reed et al.[21] The mitral portion of the procedure is done following positioning of the saphenous vein grafts, but usually the left atrium is opened early for inspection of the valve and to serve as a vent. Multiple doses of oxygenated crystalloid potassium cardioplegia are used.

We have always practiced grafting of all diseased coronary arteries. However, in the particular situation of mitral regurgitation and coronary artery disease, surrounded as it is by the urgency of operation and by the specter of low cardiac output postoperatively, frequently only the major coronary branches are grafted. Reports from the Cleveland Clinic[22] and New York Univeristy[17] attest to the fact that much of the morbidity and mortality following the operation is noncardiac. Perioperative infarction and lack of reversal of all ischemic segments, by implication, are not major factors. Therefore, a slavish dedication to "complete" revascularization may not be warranted. Clearly, however, historical and present results are improved with appropriate coronary artery bypass grafting as compared with no coronary artery bypass grafting. The report from the Cleveland Clinic, extending from 1970 to 1983 (300 patients, 7.3% mortality), failed to show any positive improvement over time in operative results. Additionally, those authors noted that patients with ischemic valve disease "without papillary muscle rupture had dismal late results." Has there been any improvement in survival over time? What are the present expectations for short- and long-term survival?

Lytle et al.,[22] DiSesa et al.,[16] Czer et al.,[15] and others have shown no improvement in expectation for early survival over time. In fact, in each of these reports, the addition of cardioplegia has not appreciably improved results (as opposed to the case of aortic valve replacement and coronary artery bypass grafting).[23, 24] Thus, historical data seem to represent present expectations. Operative mortality is between 7% and 20% and 5-year survival for mitral regurgitation–coronary artery bypass grafting is 50% to 60%.

What strategies might decrease operative risk? I suggest the following: (1) aggressive hemodynamic support before operation, including pharmacologic and mechanical unloading and vigorous inotropic intervention; (2) a policy of extended observation before operation, if possible; (3) a determined effort to avoid mitral surgery except in 3/3 regurgitation; (4) a closer look at repair as opposed to valve replacement; and (5) extended controlled reperfusion following removal of the aortic cross clamp as reported by Lazar et al.,[25] Teoh et al.,[26] and Kirklin.[27]

Unfortunately, we have identified few factors in the postoperative care period that may lead to improved survival. Obviously, a situation that preserves subsystem circulation, sustains cardiac output, and diminishes myocardial oxygen uptake is optimal. Some investigators have found norepinephrine (levarterenol) and prostaglandin E_1 beneficial. For best inotropic support in this situation, I suggest the use of amrinone.

References

1. Auscultation of the heart, in Hurst JW (ed): *The Heart*, ed 6. New York, McGraw-Hill Book Co, 1986, p 191.
2. Heikkila J: Mitral incompetence complicating acute myocardial infarction. *Br Heart J* 1967; 29:162–169.
3. Nagel RE, Walker D, Granger RG: The angiographic assessment of mitral incompetence. *Clin Radiol* 1968; 19:154.
4. Helmcke F, Nanda NC, Hsiung MC, et al: Color Doppler assessment of mitral regurgitation with orthogonal planes. *Circulation* 1987; 75:175–183.
5. Balu V, Hershowitz S, Masud ARZ, et al: Mitral regurgitation in coronary artery disease. *Chest* 1982; 81:550–555.
6. Carpentier A: Cardiac valve surgery: The "French correction." *J Thorac Cardiovasc Surg* 1983; 86:323–337.
7. Duran CG, Pomar JL, Revuelta JM, et al: Conservative operation for mitral insufficiency: Critical analysis supported by postoperative hemodynamic studies of 72 patients. *J Thorac Cardiovasc Surg* 1980; 79:326–337.
8. Bonchek LI, Olinger GN, Siegel R, et al: Left ventricular performance after mitral reconstruction for mitral regurgitation. *J Thorac Cardiovasc Surg* 1984; 88:122–127.
9. Kay GL, Kay JH, Zubiate P, et al: Mitral valve repair for mitral regurgitation secondary to coronary artery disease. *Circulation* 1986; 74:I88–I98.
10. Pinson CW, Cobanoglu A, Metzdorff MT, et al: Late surgical results for ischemic mitral regurgitation: Role of wall motion score and severity of regurgitation. *J Thorac Cardiovasc Surg* 1984; 88:663–672.
11. Salomon NW, Stinson EB, Griepp RB, et al: Patient-related risk factors as predictors of results following isolated mitral valve replacement. *Ann Thorac Surg* 1977; 24:519–530.
12. Chaffin JS, Daggett WM: Mitral valve replacement: A 9-year follow-up of risks and survivals. *Ann Thorac Surg* 1979; 27:312–319.
13. Andrade IG, Cartier R, Panisi P, et al: Factors influencing early and late survival in patients with combined mitral valve replacement and myocardial revascularization and in those with isolated replacement. *Ann Thorac Surg* 1987; 44:607–613.
14. Karp RB: Mitral valve replacement and coronary artery bypass grafting. *Ann Thorac Surg* 1982; 34:480–481.
15. Czer LSC, Gray RJ, DeRobertis MA, et al: Mitral valve replacement: Impact of coronary artery disease and determinants of prognosis after revascularization. *Circulation* 1984; 70:I198–I207.
16. DiSesa VJ, Cohn LH, Collins JJ, et al: Determinants of operative survival following combined mitral valve replacement and coronary revascularization. *Ann Thorac Surg* 1982; 34:482–489.

17. Connolly MW, Gelbfish JS, Jacobowitz IJ, et al: Surgical results for mitral regurgitation from coronary artery disease. J Thorac Cardiovasc Surg 1986; 91:379–388.
18. Kay PH, Nunley DL, Grunkemeier GL, et al: Late results of combined mitral valve replacement and coronary bypass surgery. J Am Coll Cardiol 1985; 5:29–33.
19. Magovern JA, Pennock JL, Campbell DB, et al: Risks of mitral valve replacement and mitral valve replacement with coronary artery bypass. Ann Thorac Surg 1985; 39:346–352.
20. Tepe NA, Edmunds LH: Operation for acute postinfarction mitral insufficiency and cardiogenic shock. J Thorac Cardiovasc Surg 1985; 89:525–530.
21. Reed GE, Kloth HH, Kiely B, et al: Long-term results of mitral anuloplasty in children with rheumatic mitral regurgitation. Circulation 1973; 49, 50(suppl II):189–192.
22. Lytle BW, Cosgrove DM, Gill CC, et al: Mitral valve replacement combined with myocardial revascularization: Early and late results for 300 patients, 1970 to 1983. Circulation 1985; 71:1179–1190.
23. Richardson JV, Kouchoukos NT, Wright JO, et al: Combined aortic valve replacement and myocardial revascularization: Results in 220 patients. Circulation 1979; 59:75–81.
24. Lytle BW, Cosgrove DM, Loop FD, et al: Replacement of aortic valve combined with myocardial revascularization: Determinants of early and late risk for 500 patients, 1967–1981. Circulation 1983; 68:II49–II62.
25. Lazar HL, Buckberg GD, Manganaro AM, et al: Myocardial energy replenishment and reversal of ischemic damage by substrate enhancement of secondary blood cardioplegia with amino acids during reperfusion. J Thorac Cardiovasc Surg 1980; 80:350–359.
26. Teoh KH, Christakis GT, Weisel RD, et al: Accelerated myocardial metabolic recovery with terminal warm blood cardioplegia. J Thorac Cardiovasc Surg 1986; 91:888–895.
27. Kirklin JW: Personal communication, 1987.

Reoperations for Coronary Artery Disease

Claude M. Grondin, M.D.

Head of Cardiothoracic Surgery, St. Luke's Hospital, Cleveland, Ohio

James C. Thornton, M.D.

Cardiothoracic Surgeon, St. Luke's Hospital, Cleveland, Ohio

James C. Engle, M.D.

Cardiothoracic Surgeon, St. Luke's Hospital, Cleveland, Ohio

Helmut Schreiber, M.D.

Chief of Surgery, St. Luke's Hospital, Cleveland, Ohio

Frederick S. Cross, M.D.

Cardiothoracic Surgeon, St. Luke's Hospital, Cleveland, Ohio

In 1987, over 275,000 patients underwent coronary artery bypass grafting (CABG) in the United States, more than double the figures of 1980.[1, 2] It is estimated that between 15% and 20% of patients who are subjected to CABG may require a second operation within a decade.[3, 4] The number of reoperations may have peaked, however. The age of the patients at first operation has steadily increased over the years and now approaches 65 years.[5] Ten years later, the risk of reoperation may prove prohibitive because of aging and other associated diseases. Moreover, the current widespread use of the internal mammary artery (IMA) graft may preclude the need for a second procedure. On the other hand, the majority of patients undergoing myocardial revascularization nowadays require multiple vein grafts in conjunction with the arterial graft[6]; a fair number of them may become candidates for reoperation owing to the progressive attrition rate of vein grafts. Repeated CABG carries a higher risk because of the patient's advanced age and the frequent concomitant deterioration in his left ventricular function and coronary anatomy. As the situations faced before and during operation are often of a more critical nature, reoperation also represents for the surgeon a greater challenge. The purpose of this chapter is

Adv Card Surg 1:93–110, 1990
© 1990, Year Book Medical Publishers, Inc.
0889-5074/90/01-093-110-$04.00

to review the indications and the current results of reoperation and to describe in some detail the technique of secondary revascularization.

Factors Responsible for Reoperation

Factors responsible for reoperation range from incomplete initial revascularization to progression of coronary artery disease and intrinsic graft disease. There are three periods during which reoperation may become necessary: early, within the first or second year; after 4 or 5 years have elapsed; and beyond the eighth or ninth year. There are also three basic reasons for failure. During the first few months when angina recurs or persists, it is due either to a technical fault or to a compromised graft flow (poor distal runoff or localized graft stenosis), ultimately leading to graft occlusion. Graft thrombosis may be averted through the use of platelet inhibitors, especially in grafts with limited flow.[7] On occasion, no satisfactory explanation exists for early occlusion. Four or five years after operation, recurrence of symptoms is due to progression of disease in nongrafted arteries and also to a combination of this factor and graft thrombosis or incomplete revascularization. Whether drug therapy can influence these midterm results or conditions is unknown. Late reoperation, on the other hand, becomes necessary because of graft disease that is often associated with disease in nongrafted vessels. Most reoperations performed currently are for these two reasons, since incomplete initial revascularization has become uncommon. Nearly 70% of reoperations take place 8 to 12 years after the initial procedure, and it is in this cohort of patients that the procedure is more hazardous and the results less satisfactory. Indeed, the anatomy, the collateral circulation, the left ventricular function, and, above all, the patient's age and general condition have changed, all contributing to raising the operative risk.

In essence, progression of disease either in the native circulation or in the graft itself is the major single factor leading to current reoperations. Several common factors have been isolated and serve as predictors for reoperation. In the Cleveland Clinic series, for instance, strong predictors of reoperation were, in ascending order of importance, total cholesterol level over 300 mg/dl, hypertension, incomplete revascularization, smoking, and lack of an IMA graft.[3] Interestingly, if an IMA graft had been inserted at the first operation, these factors had little influence on eventual freedom from reoperation in survivors. In the Montreal Heart Institute study, of 143 reoperations, the analysis of variance also selected total cholesterol level as the best determinant of graft atherosclerosis.[8] Smoking was the best predictor of graft thrombosis when graft atherosclerosis was excluded. Patients with late graft changes—occlusion or stenosis—had higher low-density lipoprotein cholesterol and apolipoprotein B and lower high-density lipoprotein cholesterol fractions than patients whose grafts remained intact 10 years after operation.[9] It would appear, therefore, that some of the factors believed operative in the pathogenesis of coronary artery disease also play a role in late failure of myocardial revascularization.

Prophylaxis of Recurrence

Removal of risk factors, such as by eliminating smoking, treating hypertension, and controling serum lipids by diet and medication, must be attempted. The task is enormous, but recent data suggest that the effort may be worthwhile. Although the information on smoking and hypertension is lacking, several studies have indicated a positive effect of therapeutic intervention on platelets and cholesterol.[7, 10, 11] Indeed, several trials of aspirin and dipyridamole,[7] aspirin alone,[12] and other platelet inhibitors[10] in patients after revascularization have demonstrated a significant reduction in graft occlusion rate during the first postoperative year. No one knows the effect these agents have on late graft changes as follow-up is incomplete. On the other hand, information on the effect of lowering cholesterol on graft changes is scant. Recently, the Cholesterol Lowering Atherosclerosis Study has indicated a significant decrease in graft changes within 2 years with the lowering of cholesterol level through a combination of niacin, colestid, and diet.[11] Interestingly, patients were randomized in this study at an average of 3.7 years after operation. Similarily, a randomized trial sponsored by the National Heart, Lung, and Blood Institute is currently under way that will study the effect of cholesterol-lowering agents in combination with low-dose oral anticoagulants on late graft and coronary artery changes. Therapy is to begin 1 to 7 years after CABG and angiographic follow-up to extend to 5 years after entry.

On the other hand, the best prophylaxis would appear to be the use of IMA grafts. Lytle and Loop[13] followed up a group of 1,000 patients subjected to double IMA grafts and reported that only three patients needed reoperation during a 22-month follow-up. Barner and coworkers[14] earlier underlined the lack of changes in 125 IMA grafts between 1 and 5 years after operation, and several groups have since reported patency of well over 80% at 8 to 10 years after CABG.[15–17]

Risk of Reoperation

Operative mortality for reoperation is higher than for primary revascularization procedure. It ranges from 3% to 9% (Table 1) and depends on (1) the period studied, (2) the time elapsed since the initial operation, (3) the experience of the surgeon, (4) the presence of atherosclerotic grafts, and (5) the age of the patient.[18–23] The risk of perioperative myocardial infarction (MI) is also higher because myocardial protection cannot be as adequate owing to changes in collateral as well as antegrade coronary flow. The presence of atherosclerotic grafts, on the other hand, adds to the risk be-

TABLE 1.
Risk of Reoperation (%)

Risk	Mayo Clinic[18] (n = 106)	Cleveland Clinic[23] (n = 1,500)	Texas[22] (n = 958)	Stanford[20] (n = 71)
	Series			
Operative mortality	2.8	3.4	9.2	2.8
Perioperative MI	7.5	7.2	—	14
Reentry for bleeding	4.7	6.8	—	0
Wound infection	1.9	1.6	—	3
Neurologic deficit	0.9	2.1	—	—

cause of the potential for intraoperative embolization of graft debris. In recent large series, the incidence of preoperative MI ranges from 8% to 14%.[21, 23] Other perioperative complications add to the list: postoperative bleeding requiring reentry is around 10%,[23] and neurologic complications (2%) are more frequent as the age of the patient increases. Wound infection does not appear to be more frequent following reoperations.[13] Hence, the risk of reoperation is higher mainly because in-hospital mortality and postoperative MI—the two major end points—occur with greater frequency than in primary revascularization procedures. The other complications, on the other hand, although slightly higher in certain instances, appear to be encountered with an acceptable frequency. With accumulated experience, the incidence of perioperative MI and death has decreased appreciably in large series.[21, 22] This is due in great part to improvement in surgical technique and better understanding of the intraoperative conditions and risk.

Late Results of Reoperation

Although operative mortality, early survival, and symptomatic relief[24] after revascularization may equal those recorded following primary operations, it is apparent that mid- and long-term (5- to 10-year) results are not as satisfactory[18, 20, 23] (Table 2). Thus, in the Mayo Clinic Series,[18] the percentage of patients free of cardiac event at 5 and 7 years was 28% and 26%, respectively (63% at each interval of follow-up if mild angina was excluded). Only 28% of patients were asymptomatic at 5 years. In the Cleveland Clinic's most recent study,[23] on the other hand, survival at 5 and 10 years was 90% and 75%, compared with 94% and 89% in the Mayo series at 5 and 7 years, and the percentage of patients free of cardiac event was 76% and 48% at mid- and long-term follow-up. Conversely, 52% of the Cleveland series' patients were asymptomatic at 5 years, while in the

TABLE 2.
Late Results of Reoperation

Results	Series			
	Mayo Clinic[18] (n = 106)	Cleveland Clinic[23] (n = 1,500)	Texas[22] (n = 958)	Stanford[20] (n = 71)
Survival				
5 yr	94	90	80	—
10 yr	89*	75	58	—
Event free				
5 yr	63†	76	—	—
10 yr	26*	48	—	—
Asymptomatic				
5 yr	28	52	—	31‡

*At 7 years.
†Free of class III-IV angina.
‡At 2.2 years.

Stanford series[20] the percentage of patients free of symptoms (31%) paralleled that of the patients in the Mayo study.

The reasons for the discrepancy noted in these various studies are not readily apparent. Two series contained a comparatively small number of patients[18, 20] and preceded the larger series at variance in terms of overall results[23] by 4 and 9 years, respectively. Better long-term results may have been due to greater use of the IMA during reoperation (>50%) in the more recent and larger series and, perhaps, from the attainment of a more complete revascularization. Complete revascularization has many meanings, however, and often this parameter cannot be used as a common denominator. Be that as it may, most authors agree on the concept that reoperation may be accomplished with low mortality and morbidity and that the potential for long-term benefit is realized in the majority of patients.

Surgical Technique

General Approach

Myocardial revascularization differs on the second attempt primarily because the anatomy changes with time. It is apparent, also, that the technique varies from one surgeon to another. Variation according to the time frame makes sense: the operative findings are not the same 10 days after operation, when, for instance, adhesions are loose and not yet vascular, compared with 6 weeks later, when they bleed easily. Further, in the early postoperative years, grafts may be handled in no specific manner, whereas 10 years after operation, they may be filled with atheromatous material and need to be manipulated with the utmost care. That the technique varies from one center to another remains somewhat of a mystery because of our conviction that the second operation need not be approached differently, although, admittedly, it is more tedious and requires a more patient dissection.

Some recommend the right lateral thoracic approach when only the circumflex artery is involved[25], others readily enter both pleural cavities following a midline sternotomy and approach the intrapericardial structures from each side. Further, several surgeons employ an oscillating orthopedic saw during the second sternotomy to cut the outer table first and, gingerly, the inner table while retracting the superficial layer.[13] All of these variations aim at avoiding accidental entry into the cardiac chambers or catastrophic laceration of patent grafts[26] or, simply, at circumventing the task of taking down adhesions. These refinements, although ingenious, may be superfluous as the difficulty of reentry may be tackled head on (see below).

Anesthesia differs little for reoperation. Before induction, a catheter is introduced in the radial artery and a Swan-Ganz floating catheter is positioned in the pulmonary artery via the internal jugular vein or, on occasion, the subclavian vein. Intravenous nitroglycerine administration is begun once the cardiac output and systemic vascular resistance are obtained. Anesthesia is slowly induced with fentanyl-morphine in combination, and the trachea is intubated. Cardiac output and arterial blood gases are measured again while the patient's skin is prepared with iodine solution. Both legs are prepared circumferentially, as usual, to gain access to either the long or short saphenous veins. Dissection of the groin for possible femoral cannulation is rarely carried out.

Reopening of the Sternum Early After Operation

During the first month after operation, the simple removal of the sternal wires suffices to reenter the mediastinum and finger dissection to free the heart from its loose adhesions to the anterior thorax. Adhesions are loose and bleed little in the early postoperative period, making reexploration nonhazardous. By the second or third week, adhesions are stronger and bleed easily, and target vessels have become less apparent. The period extending from the third or fourth week to the third or fourth month, on the other hand, represents the riskiest window: the sternum has begun to heal, the heart remains swollen, and adhesions have stiffened. The sternum is opened then in the same manner as a reoperation conducted years later; the sternal edges must not be spread laterally but, rather, must be lifted vertically with the help of a rake or a Favaloro-type retractor. Rupture or tear of the anterior right ventricular (RV) wall is more often due to adhesion of the RV to the sternal edges, which, when spread laterally, can shear the thin ventricle. When the sternum is lifted up via the Favaloro retractor, the cardiac structures, by gravity, are pulled away from the anterior chest wall, and adhesions may be severed with the electrocautery device. Sharp dissection with the cautery or the scissors is used at all times: blunt dissection is to be avoided.

Resternotomy Late After Operation

Beyond the first 6 months, resternotomy is approached in precisely the same manner as for primary sternotomy. The skin and soft tissues are incised and the periosteum is cut with the electrocautery. The xyphoid process is incised with curved scissors along with the first 1 or 2 cm of lower sternum until bone marrow is seen. No blunt dissection with the finger or other instruments above the sternal notch or below the lower sternum is carried out. As for the first operation, a standard sternal saw is used and is held in an axis perpendicular to that of the sternum. Beforehand, the operating table is lowered to its lowest point and the base of the saw held firmly against the underside of the sternum so as to literally lift the patient from the table (Fig 1). This step allows the mediastinal structures to move away by gravity and ensures intimal contact of the foot of the base of the saw with the inner sternal table. The saw is maneuvered slowly and firmly upward and is tipped slightly next to the manubrium so that its axis remains perpendicular to the sternum. No attempt is made to spread the edges of the sternum; rather, the left half of the xyphoid process or lower sternum is lifted (that is, at a point well below the inferior border of the right side of the heart) with the Favaloro retractor (Fig 2). A slight twist of the knob will lift the lower sternum enough to dissect with the cautery and push the right side of the heart down. As the mediastinal structures drop down, the marginal border of the right side of the heart and the junction of the right side of the heart and diaphragm are uncovered. A plane of dissection is usually found leading to free pericardial spaces overlying the diaphragm. Dissection is further extended above and to the left until the area beyond the left anterior descending artery (LAD) is encountered or a graft (vein or IMA) to the LAD is identified. The aorta and the pulmonary artery come next into view. No further dissection of the left structures is necessary, and the Favaloro retractor is removed and placed in the same area on the opposite side next to the xyphoid process for the freeing of the right atrium, the vena cava, and the right half of the ascending aorta.

The pericardial edge is located close to the diaphragm; often, blunt dissection may be used on the right atrium and the superior vena cava—ascending aorta junction. When grafts are present and still patent—diseased or not—dissection is terminated at that point and the standard sternal retractor replaces the Favaloro. Heparin is administered through the right atrium, and double purse-string sutures are applied onto the atrium (for single cannulation) and the ascending aorta. Cardiopulmonary bypass is instituted, and the remainder of the aorta and pulmonary artery are freed to allow eventual placement of a cross clamp. When an IMA graft is present, this may prove tedious (see below).

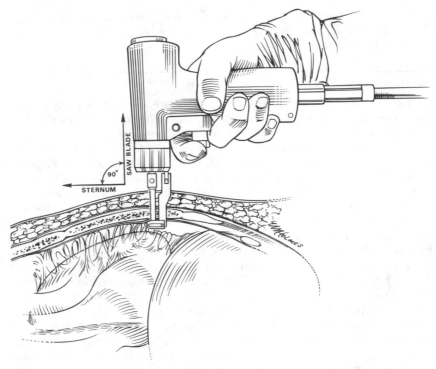

FIG 1.
Illustration of standard sternal saw used in reoperations. Holding the tip of the saw parallel to underside of lower sternum and the axis of the saw at a right angle with the sternum, the surgeon pushes the saw in a cephalad direction while literally lifting the patient off the table. This keeps the blunt tip of the saw in close apposition to the inner sternal table while the mediastinal structures fall down by gravity.

Reoperation in the Presence of Patent Grafts

A second pitfall encountered in late reoperations is the presence of patent grafts, be they an IMA or a saphenous vein graft, especially if the venous graft is diseased. Accidental transection of a patent graft on one hand may lead to acute ischemia occurring quite distant in time from cannulation and cardiopulmonary bypass, and, on the other, undue manipulation of an atherosclerotic graft may result in an equally catastrophic ischemic event. Vein grafts rarely cross the midline en route to their target vessels, but long IMA grafts may lie close to the midline in the case of a left IMA (LIMA) to LAD graft or actually cross over in the case of the right IMA to LAD graft.[27] Diseased vein grafts or any apparently sane graft in place for more than 8 or 9 years should not be handled: eventually, it should be replaced after early ligation, after cross-clamping of the aorta.[4] The IMA graft, on the other hand, in its usual LIMA-LAD position, is dissected once cardiopul-

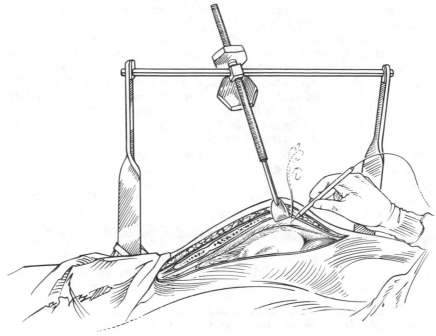

FIG 2.
Favaloro retractor (single fork) inserted under xyphoid-sternal junction, lifting the chest away from the right ventricle. The electrocautery frees the adhesions underneath the sternum.

monary bypass has begun. The pedicle is usually very adherent to the left upper mediastinum next to the pulmonary artery, and it is virtually impossible to identify the mammary artery itself except near the anastomosis, where tails of old nonabsorbable sutures may be seen. The IMA pedicle must be freed from the pulmonary artery to avoid trauma during cross-clamping of the aorta; the pedicle itself also needs to be clamped during cardioplegic infusion to prevent myocardial rewarming.

Often, the IMA graft gets in the way of a newly constructed circumflex artery graft when the latter is brought anterior to the graft vessels for proximal anastomosis. Under these circumstances, the graft may be allowed to course posterior to the pedicle to avoid kinking or angulation. It may also be brought behind the great vessels through the transverse sinus for anastomosis to the right side of the aorta or, on occasion, behind the heart to the right side, over the right atrium, and onto the right side of the aorta. This requires a longer vein segment and benefits from the passage behind the inferior vena cava en route to the aorta. On the other hand, passing through the transverse sinus in reoperation may be hazardous, especially when an old graft courses through it. Another option is to bring the new vein graft anterior to the pedicle on the left side and hook it to the aorta head on without beveling its end so that the graft may hop over the IMA pedicle without angulation (Fig 3).

Atherosclerotic grafts represent the most serious pitfall. Dissection of the heart should be limited to the right ventricle, the ascending aorta, and the right atrium near the appendiceal remnant. Once the aorta is clamped, all diseased grafts are transected near the aorta and allowed to empty their content with the initial gush of cardioplegic fluid mixed with blood. When return is clear, the grafts are tied off. They are then transected near the distal anastomosis and through each cardioplegic infusion allowed to back bleed to flush distal debris (Fig 4). When the coronary anastomosis is completed, the distal end of the old vein graft may be tied with a large clip or a stick tie. Segments of the old grafts are sent for microscopic study. At times it may be necessary and practical to use the distal short stump of a cleaned graft as a site for additional cardioplegic infusion (Fig 5). This may be repeated and of critical benefit in the case of a newly constructed IMA graft when cardioplegic infusion from the ascending aorta cannot reach that particular territory because of total flow dependence on the previous graft. When inserting several new grafts, it is wise to start with the most strategic one and use the new graft, if not an IMA graft, for cardioplegic infusion. When an IMA graft is inserted, the old vein stump may be utilized for infusion.

Cardioplegic Infusion, Handling of Old Grafts, and Proximal Anastomosis

Infusion of cardioplegic solution requires planning during reoperation.[4] When all grafts are closed, no special precautions are needed: the operation is performed in the same manner as for any primary revascularization procedure. In the case of open grafts, graft flow, by necessity, is interrupted either through clamping of the aorta (or of the graft itself in the case of an IMA graft) or through transection of disease grafts. Cardioplegic solutions may not reach arterial beds distal to the clamped or transected grafts. Therefore, larger amounts of solution must be used. Myocardial temperature probes are inserted and infusion is continued until temperature drops below 15° C in the critical area. Usually, 1,500 mL are required to reach this level. Subsequently, the newly constructed graft is utilized for the administration of additional solution. If an IMA graft is planned for the LAD area, the old distal stump may be used for cardioplegic infusion, and the IMA-LAD graft is fashioned last. After each distal vein graft anastomosis, cardioplegic solution is administered through the graft only if there is no preoperative evidence of antegrade flow to the area via the native circulation. At least 500 mL are injected into the ascending aorta, and an additional 100 to 150 mL are pushed through each new graft as needed before the next anastomosis.

Performance of the proximal anastomosis must also be planned. If no IMA graft is present or planned, all proximal aortic anastomoses are performed under the same aortic clamping using one final aortic infusion following the last distal anastomosis. When an IMA graft is present, especially

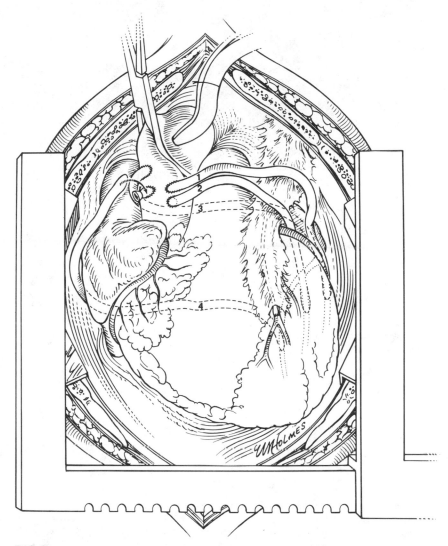

FIG 3.

Portrayal of various routes a newly constructed graft to circumflex may take in the presence of a patent internal mammary artery (old) graft: anterior to the pedicle *(1),* with the potential for kinking distally; anterior or posterior to the pedicle *(2),* with the anastomosis direct and not tangential to the aorta; behind the great vessels *(3);* and, finally, behind the heart, to the right, underneath the inferior vena cava, and onto the aorta *(4).*

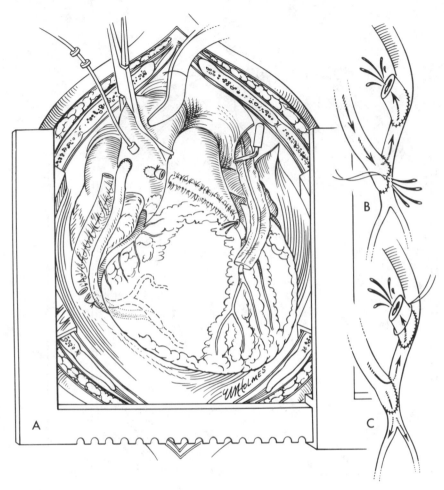

FIG 4.
Both old grafts to left anterior descending artery (LAD) and right coronary artery
(RCA) transected and tied are replaced by left internal mammary artery–LAD graft
and vein graft to RCA **(A).** Proximal anastomosis of RCA graft fashioned on old
aortic site and with the aorta clamped if no flow exists preoperatively via collateral
or native circulation. Internal mammary artery graft should remain clamped while
aorta is clamped. Insert **(B** and **C)** shows flushing of blood or cardioplegic fluid
through distal anastomosis while stump of old graft remains untied to allow debris
to be flushed out. All proximal stumps have been tied following transection and
initial flushing from cardioplegic infusion into ascending aorta.

to the LAD, the aorta and the IMA pedicle may be unclamped and the
proximal anastomosis performed in the customary manner. When more
than one aortic anastomosis is needed and no antegrade flow is known to
exist distal to the new grafts, it is best to leave the aorta and the IMA graft
(if present) clamped during the performance of the aortic anastomoses.

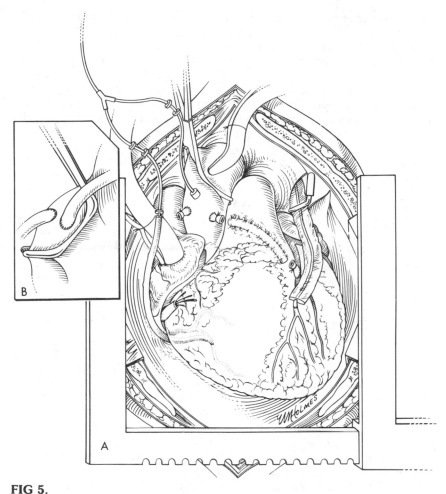

FIG 5.
A, drawing of newly constructed vein graft to right coronary artery (RCA) and internal mammary artery (IMA) graft to left anterior descending artery (planned graft to circumflex not displayed). Cardioplegic infusion is through ascending aorta and newly constructed graft to RCA (IMA graft should be clamped all through the aortic cross clamping). Inset **(B)** shows aortic anastomoses constructed on old sites with virtually no remnant (2-mm cuff) of old grafts.

Recent studies suggest that myocardial function is better preserved when all distal and proximal anastomoses are done under one clamping during primary revascularization.[28] At times, in the presence of a patent IMA graft, the aorta may be unclamped and the aortic anastomosis of a venous graft to a jeopardized territory constructed rapidly, and the side clamp removed and reapplied for anastomosis of noncritical grafts. This option should not be taken when no antegrade native flow is known to exist to the territory revascularized by vein conduits.

Early clamping of the aorta and transection-ligation of all atherosclerotic grafts have been the subject of debate. This step was suggested[29] to avoid embolization of debris during cardioplegic infusion since the fluid characteristics of the infusion (pressure, nonpulsatile flow, low viscosity and temperature) differ considerably from normal coronary flow. No doubt, embolization occurs mainly during dissection through graft manipulation.[4] Some grafts are literally filled with what has been termed "toothpaste atheroma," and graft transection at both ends followed by flushing and ligation represent the only safe method. Some surgeons[13] use a first injection through the ascending aorta—hence, through the old grafts—and, subsequently, transect the grafts. In the presence of severely diseased grafts, this compromise may prove hazardous. The objection that cardioplegia and cooling will not take place through a limited native circulation has not proved valid in our experience. All hearts have paralyzed, and areas distal to ligated grafts have reached a temperature below 15° C with increased infusion despite a severely restricted native circulation. It is our belief that major ischemia occurs either during the dissection of the heart and manipulation of the diseased grafts or during the performance of the aortic anastomoses when the aorta is unclamped and the heart, inevitably, is rewarming.

When to Ligate Diseased Vein Grafts?

Intraoperative atheroembolism from diseased grafts was alluded to by Thomas and colleagues[30] in the 1970s. Later, following postmortem demonstration of intracoronary atheroemboli, Keon and coworkers[29] suggested graft ligation. More recently,[4] we proposed transection of all grafts before cardioplegic infusion and noted in a subsequent report[21] its efficacy in patients who had at least one diseased graft 9 years or more after operation. Others have suggested an earlier schedule for replacement of all grafts in patients reoperated on 5 years after initial revascularization whose angiogram demonstrates at least one diseased graft.[31]

Graft disease may have an early histologic onset. A recent large study conducted at 1 and 5 years after operation revealed that 40% of grafts showed changes on the late angiogram.[32] Operative mortality may reach 10% to 15% and the incidence of perioperative MI may be as high as 25% in subsets of patients with patent atherosclerotic grafts subjected to reoperation.[21] Graft disease may involve 75% of grafts at 10 to 12 years and with time all grafts.[33] Therefore, removing all grafts beyond 8 or 9 years, even those that appear free of disease, may be a logical policy. When replacement is possible by an IMA graft, perhaps it should be extended to patients reoperated on only 5 years after initial revascularization. The replacement of an (apparently) disease-free graft by a venous conduit would offer limited protection since the individual, in this case, already has demonstrated a propensity for early graft disease. This dilemma may be considerably lessened if some degree of protection from atheromatous degeneration can be obtained through platelet inhibitors and cholesterol-lowering agents.

Follow-up of Patients After Primary Revascularization: When to Operate?

Recurrence of angina or MI usually constitutes the main indication for angiographic evaluation and reoperation in most series. Myocardial infarction that occurs late after CABG usually involves a small area in comparison with a conventional MI.[34] Patients who present recurrent angina, on the other hand, often exhibit an unstable syndrome. Anxiety over recurrent disease probably plays a major role in this instance. On occasion, patients will be subjected on their yearly postoperative visit to an exercise test that reveals changes previously undetected. In some instances, a coronary arteriogram is requested 8 or 10 years after operation as part of research protocol or at the request of the referring physician or even the patient. Such a study may well show progression of coronary and/or graft disease. This, in turn, gives rise to a dilemma of proportion: What is the proper form of treatment for asymptomatic coronary or graft disease? If, on one hand, there is no significant graft disease, but significant coronary artery disease in nongrafted vessels, reoperation is based on the exercise test and if doubt persists on a thallium perfusion study. On the other hand, if significant graft disease is present and involves an important area of myocardium with or without associated native coronary artery disease, reoperation is advocated provided there are no contraindications to reoperation such as debilitating diseases or conditions limiting the patient's life expectancy. Current standards of follow-up of patients with vein bypass grafts beyond the fifth year should include exercise tests, noninvasive perfusion scans, and, beyond 10 years, a repeated coronary arteriogram.

Summary

Coronary reoperations have come of age. As many as 40,000 such operations are performed annually in the United States. Mortality and morbidity now approach those of primary revascularization. In certain groups of patients, however, operative mortality and perioperative complications remain high. Long-term results probably cannot match those of primary operation because revascularization and myocardial protection are not as complete, preoperative left ventricular function is not as intact, and, above all, the patient is not as young and in as good condition as for the first procedure. Nevertheless, freedom from serious cardiac events is expected in 50% to 75% of patients 5 years after reoperation. The operative risks have decreased in the past decade as predictors have been identified and technical progress has been made.

In essence, preoperative preparation, anesthetic management, and reentry are carried out in the same manner, and, when all grafts are closed, myocardial protection and the overall conduct of the operation are similar to those used during a primary procedure. The presence of a patent IMA graft provides a challenge to the surgeon as its course may unexpectedly take it behind the sternum (not all IMA grafts are taken down with metallic clips that help identify their track). An IMA graft must be clamped during cardioplegic infusion and may hinder the passage of a newly constructed graft to the circumflex artery. Open atherosclerotic grafts must not be manipulated and should be tied promptly following aortic clamping. Beyond 8 or 10 years, all vein grafts should be replaced if one is known to show advanced disease on the preoperative angiogram. The exception to this rule is uncommon but may exist: during a long and eventful procedure, the surgeon may feel that additional grafting would jeopardize the immediate outcome of the patient. Under those circumstances, he should abstain, to be sure. No doubt, reoperation late after revascularization represents a challenge. However, the rewards far outweigh the pitfalls in most instances.

Whether current intervention on risk factors and drug therapy will help arrest the progression of coronary artery disease or prevent graft disease remains to be seen. It appears that the maximal use of the IMA during primary operations represents the most important single step and its use during reoperation may ensure improved long-term results.

References

1. Bourassa MG, Alderman EL, Bertrand M, et al: Report of the Joint ISFC/WHO Taskforce on Coronary Angioplasty. *Circulation* 1988; 78:780–789.
2. National Center for Health Statistics: *1986 Summary: National Hospital Discharge Survey,* Dept of Health and Human Services publication (PHS) 87-1250. Hyattsville, Md, National Center for Health Statistics, Public Health Service, 1987.
3. Cosgrove DM, Loop FD, Lytle BW, et al: Predictors of reoperation after myocardial revascularization. *J Thorac Cardiovasc Surg* 1986; 92:811–821.
4. Grondin CM, Pomar JL, Hebert Y, et al: Reoperation in patients with patent atherosclerotic coronary vein grafts: A different approach to a different disease. *J Thorac Cardiovasc Surg* 1984; 87:379–385.
5. Naunheim KS, Flore AC, Wadley JJ, et al: The changing profile of the patient undergoing coronary artery bypass surgery. *J Am Coll Cardiol* 1988; 11:494–498.
6. Grondin CM, Campeau L, Thornton JC, et al: Coronary artery bypass grafting with saphenous vein. *Circulation* 1989; 79(suppl I):1–6.
7. Cheseboro JH, Clements IP, Fuster V, et al: A platelet inhibitor drug trial in coronary-artery bypass operations. *N Engl J Med* 1982; 307:73–78.
8. Solymoss BC, Nadeau P, Campeau L, et al: Late thrombosis of saphenous vein coronary bypass related to risk factors. *Circulation* 1988; 78(suppl 2):140–143.
9. Campeau L, Enjalbert M, Lesperance J, et al: The relation of risk factors to the development of atherosclerosis in saphenous-vein bypass grafts and the progression of disease in the native circulation: A study 10 years after aortocoronary bypass surgery. *N Engl J Med* 1984; 311:1329–1332.
10. Limet R, David JL, Magotteaux P, et al: Prevention of aorto-coronary bypass

graft occlusion: Beneficial effect of ticlopidine on early and late patency rates of venous coronary bypass grafts: A double-blind study. *J Thorac Cardiovasc Surg* 1987; 94:773–783.

11. Blackenhorn DH, Nessim SA, Johnson RL, et al: Beneficial effects of combined colestipol-niacin therapy on coronary atherosclerosis and coronary venous bypass grafts. *JAMA* 1987; 257:3233–3240.

12. Gitler B, Gitler ES: Efficacy of antiplatelet drugs in the maintenance of aorto-coronary vein bypass graft patency. *Am Heart J* 1983; 106:563–570.

13. Lytle BW, Loop FD: Coronary reoperations. *Surg Clin North Am* 1988; 68:559–580.

14. Barner HB, Swartz MT, Mudd JG, et al: Late patency of the internal mammary artery as a coronary bypass conduit. *Ann Thorac Surg* 1982; 34:408–412.

15. Grondin CM, Campeau L, Lesperance J, et al: Comparison of late changes in internal mammary artery and saphenous vein grafts in two consecutive series of patients 10 years after operation. *Circulation* 1984; 70(suppl 1):208–212.

16. Okies JE, Page US, Bigelow JC, et al: The left internal mammary artery: The graft of choice. *Circulation* 1984; 70(suppl 1):213–221.

17. Lytle BW, Loop FD, Cosgrove DM, et al: Long-term (5 to 12 years) serial studies of internal mammary artery and saphenous vein coronary bypass grafts. *J Thorac Cardiovasc Surg* 1985; 89:248–258.

18. Schaff HV, Orszulak TA, Gersh BJ, et al: The morbidity and mortality of reoperation for coronary artery disease and analysis of late results with use of actuarial estimate of even-free survival. *J Thorac Cardiovasc Surg* 1983; 85:508–515.

19. Foster ED, Fisher LD, Kaiser GC, et al: Comparison of operative mortality and morbidity for initial and repeat coronary artery bypass grafting: The Coronary Artery Surgery Study (CASS) registry experience. *Ann Thorac Surg* 1984; 38:563–570.

20. Allen RH, Stinson EB, Oyer PE, et al: Predictive variables in reoperation for coronary artery disease. *J Thorac Cardiovasc Surg* 1978; 75:186–192.

21. Grondin CM: Reoperation in patients with coronary graft disease, in McGoon DC (ed): *Cardiac Surgery*, ed 2. Philadelphia, FA Davis Co, 1987, pp 31–39.

22. Hall RJ, Elayda MA, Gray AG, et al: Reoperation for coronary artery disease, abstracted. *J Am Coll Cardiol* 1986; 7:32A.

23. Lytle BW, Loop FD, Cosgrove DM, et al: Fifteen hundred coronary reoperations: Results and determinants of early and late survival. *J Thorac Cardiovasc Surg* 1987; 93:847–859.

24. Vouhe P, Grondin CM: Reoperation for coronary graft failure: Clinical and angiographic results in 43 patients. *Ann Thorac Surg* 1979; 27:328–334.

25. Ungerleider RM, Mills NL, Wechsler AS: Left thoracotomy for reoperation coronary artery bypass procedures. *Ann Thorac Surg* 1985; 40:11–15.

26. Loop FD: Catastrophic hemorrhage during sternal reentry, editorial. *Ann Thorac Surg* 1984; 37:271–272.

27. Baillot RG, Loop FD, Cosgrove DM, et al: Reoperation after previous grafting with the internal mammary artery: Technique and early results. *Ann Thorac Surg* 1985; 40:271–273.

28. Weisel RD, Hoy FBY, Baird RJ, et al: A comparison of alternative cardioplegic techniques. *J Thorac Cardiovasc Surg* 1983; 86:97–107.

29. Keon WJ, Heggtveit HA, Leduc J: Perioperative myocardial infarction caused by atheroembolism. *J Thorac Cardiovasc Surg* 1982; 84:849–855.

30. Thomas CS, Alford WC, Burrus GR, et al: Results of reoperation for failed aortocoronary bypass grafts. Arch Surg 1976; 111:1210–1213.
31. Marshall WB, Saffitz J, Kouchoukos NT: Management during reoperation of aortocoronary saphenous vein grafts with minimal atherosclerosis by angiography. Ann Thorac Surg 1986; 42:163–167.
32. Fitzgibbon GM, Leach AJ, Keon WJ, et al: Coronary bypass graft fate: Angiographic study of 1,179 vein grafts early, 1 year and 5 years after operation. J Thorac Cardiovasc Surg 1986; 91:773–778.
33. Grondin CM: Graft disease in patients with coronary bypass grafting: Why does it start? Where do we stop? editorial. J Thorac Cardiovasc Surg 1986; 92:323–329.
34. Crean PA, Waters DD, Bosch X, et al: Angiographic findings after myocardial infarction in patients with previous bypass surgery: Explanation for smaller infarcts in this group compared with control patients. Circulation 1985; 71:693–698.

Modified Fontan Procedure

Gary S. Haas, M.D.

Assistant Professor, Department of Cardiothoracic Surgery, UCLA Medical Center, Los Angeles, California

Hillel Laks, M.D.

Professor and Chief, Division of Cardiothoracic Surgery, Director, Heart Transplant Program, UCLA Medical Center, Los Angeles, California

Jeffrey M. Pearl, M.D.

Resident in Surgery, UCLA Medical Center, Los Angeles, California

Modified Fontan procedures are carried out in patients with a single ventricular chamber to separate the systemic and pulmonary venous return and to create a passive, direct connection between the systemic venous return and the pulmonary arteries. The cardiac anatomy that is created consists of a three-chambered heart with the right atrium and, in some situations, hypoplastic right ventricle, serving primarily as a nonfunctional conduit to divert systemic venous return directly to the pulmonary circulation and away from the functional ventricle. The physiological benefits of these operations include the relief of cyanosis and the alleviation of ventricular volume overload. However, patients undergoing such procedures share the common physiologic alteration in which the systemic venous pressure increases to become the principal driving force for both pulmonary blood flow and ventricular filling. Early application and experience with these procedures was limited to patients with tricuspid atresia. Subsequently, additional modifications have allowed its use in a wide spectrum of complex congenital cardiac malformations. Better understanding of this physiologic state, technical advances in the performance of the procedures, and better preoperative and postoperative patient management have significantly improved the results of this challenging operation.

Background

Natural History of the "Single Ventricle"

The original Fontan and subsequent modified Fontan procedures were developed for use in patients with a single functional ventricular component.

The natural history of these patients is generally poor and initially varies according to the amount of pulmonary blood flow.[1-3] A few patients with limited but adequate pulmonary blood flow remain stable through early childhood as long as the origin of pulmonary blood flow does not become restrictive[3]; in most, however, pulmonary blood flow does not become restrictive.[3] Most patients, however, have pulmonary blood flow that initially is usually either inadequate or excessive.[1, 2, 4-7] Patients with inadequate pulmonary blood flow develop progressive cyanosis and die of hypoxia or other related complications[6, 7]; those with excessive pulmonary blood flow develop congestive heart failure and die of either ventricular decompensation or subsequent pulmonary vascular disease.[1, 2, 5-7]

Palliative Procedures

The application of palliative procedures has markedly improved the early survival of these patients.[8] Shunting of some of the systemic circulation to the pulmonary circulation (e.g., the Blalock-Taussig operation, developed in 1945,[9] the Potts operation in 1946,[10] and the Waterston operation in 1962[11]) has provided effective palliation for restricted pulmonary blood flow.[8, 12-14] Similarly, pulmonary artery banding, as reported by Muller and Damman[15] in 1952, has provided effective palliation for unrestricted pulmonary blood flow.

Long-term results of these pallitative procedures, however, reveal increasing late mortality due to progression of subpulmonary or subaortic obstruction,[16] increasing cyanosis due to progressive narrowing systemic to pulmonary shunts, and over time, deterioration of ventricular function as a result of chronic volume overload.[3, 5, 8, 12, 14, 17] Five-year survival has been reported to be 85% for palliation of univentricular heart at the University of Alabama.[14] Ten-year survival after shunting has been reported at 72%, and 20-year survival at 50%.[12] Similarly, 15-year survival after palliation of tricuspid atresia has been reported at 50% to 70%.[2, 18-21] A poorer prognosis after all types of palliation of univentricular heart was reported by Moodie et al.,[8] who noted 10-year survival of 70% for patients with a single ventricle with "left ventricle" morphologic features, and only 25% for patients with other types of single ventricle. In addition, 49% of surviving patients in this report were limited to New York Heart Association (NYHA) functional classes III and IV.

Partial Venous Bypass

The partial diversion of caval blood directly to the pulmonary arteries, bypassing the ventricle, was introduced experimentally by Carlon et al.[22] in 1951 and by Glenn and Patino[23] in 1954. Subsequent clinical use was reported by Glenn[24] in 1958 and by Bakulev and Kolesnikov[25] in 1959. Excellent palliation has been obtained with anastomosis of the superior vena cava to the right pulmonary artery (Glenn operation), particularly when combined with a left-to-right shunt in patients older than 6 months. Ten-year survival is reported at 85%.[20, 26-28] Although uncommon, there are reports of associated complications. These include decreased right-sided pulmonary blood flow, probably related to rising hematocrit and the development of venous collateral vessels around the ligated vena cava; excessive superior vena cava pressure and superior vena cava syndrome, which are usually secondary to excessive fluid administration or elevated pulmonary vascular resistance; and pulmonary arteriovenous fistulas, which are usually confined to the right lower lobe.[27-30] Advantages of this approach include the technical ease of the shunt construction, the gratifying immediate results, and the benefits of directing venous return directly to the lung, thus increasing the gradient for oxygen transfer, avoiding the volume load on the heart, and reducing the risk for pulmonary vascular disease.[31]

Complete Venous Bypass

The promising results of partial diversion of the systemic venous blood to the pulmonary circulation encouraged efforts to achieve complete surgical correction of lesions with a single functional ventricular component by "total" diversion of the systemic venous blood to the pulmonary circulation. Early studies by Starr et al.[32] in 1943 demonstrated that the canine right ventricle could be rendered nonfunctional without causing excessive increases in venous pressure; and Robard and Wagner[33] in 1949 demonstrated bypass of the right ventricle. In classic experiments carried out in 1954 by Warden et al.,[34] staged ligation of the tricuspid valve and anastomosis of the right atrial appendage to the pulmonary artery led to successful complete diversion of systemic venous blood away from the right ventricle, and directly to the pulmonary circulation. Additional laboratory studies by Robicsek et al.[35] in 1956, Haller et al.[36] in 1966, and Just-Viera et al.[37] in 1971 confirmed the observation that exclusion of the right ventricle from the normal circulation could be well tolerated.

The early clinical experience of Hurwitt et al.[38] and Shumaker,[39] reported in 1955, with right ventricular bypass accomplished by anastomosis of the atrial appendage to the pulmonary artery, was promising; however, neither patient survived. Similar was the experience of Harrison,[40] reported in 1962, with staged atrial pulmonary anastomosis and closure of an atrial septal defect. In 1971, Fontan et al.[41, 42] reported the first successful experience with atriopulmonary shunting to treat tricuspid atresia using a technique (Fig 1) in which the transected distal right pulmonary artery was anastomosed to the superior vena cava (as in a classic Glenn operation) and the transected proximal end was connected to the right atrium with a valved aortic homograft. The atrial septal defect was closed directly, and a second homograft valve was placed at the orifice of the inferior vena cava. Kreutzer et al.[46] successfully performed operations for complete diversion of systemic venous to pulmonary circulation in two patients with

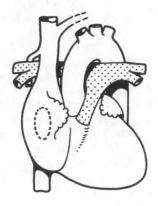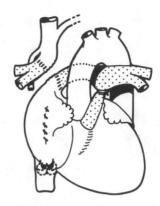

FIG 1.
A diagram of Fontan's original procedure for tricuspid atresia. The procedure included closure of the atrial septal defect, a classical Glenn shunt, and placement of a valved homograft from the right atrium to the left pulmonary artery. An additional valve was placed at the oriface of the inferior vena cava and the main pulmonary artery was ligated. (From Fontan F, Baudet E: Surgical repair of tricuspid atresia. *Thorax* 1971; 26:240. Used by permission.)

tricuspid atresia without using an inferior vena cava valve, by separating the main pulmonary artery and valve from the right ventricular outflow and anastomosing them to the right atrial appendage (Fig 2).

Subsequent experience with similar procedures, using homograft valves, reported by Ross and Somerville[43] in 1973, Stanford et al.[44] in 1973, and Miller et al.[45] in 1974, also produced survivors. Multiple additional methods have subsequently been used for valveless atriopulmonary connections (Figs 3 and 4).[56]

Modifications of the Fontan Procedure

Since these early experiences many important modifications have been made to the original Fontan procedure. Better understanding of the nature of systemic venous–pulmonary perfusion and the application of this concept to more varied and complex lesions have led to the evolution of further technical advances and refinements in the methods of isolating the systemic venous return and creating the atriopulmonary connection.

Incorporation of a hypoplastic right ventricle into the atriopulmonary connection was an important early modification. In 1978 Bowman et al.[47] reported the closure of a ventricular septal defect and placement of a valved conduit from the right atrium to a hypoplastic right ventricle for correction of tricuspid atresia. In 1979 Bjork et al.[48] reported successful inclusion of a diminutive right ventricle in an atriopulmonary connection, which in combination with a Glenn operation and closure of a ventricular septal defect accomplished complete repair of tricuspid atresia without the use of a conduit or a prosthetic valve.

The implantation of prosthetic or homograft valves within the orifice of

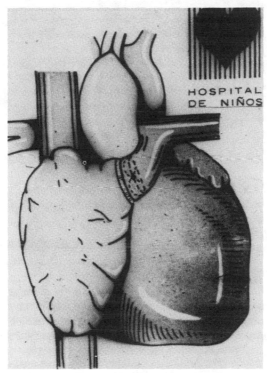

FIG 2.
The anterior atriopulmonary connection described by Kreutzer et al. The pulmonary valve was preserved within the main pulmonary artery which was attached directly to the right atrial appendage. The atrial septal defect was closed and no additional valve was inserted in the inferior venacaval oriface. (From Kreutzer G, Galíndez E, Bono H, et al: An operation for the correction of tricuspid atresia. *J Thorac Cardiovasc Surg* 1973; 66:613. Used by permission.)

the inferior vena cava was abandoned, and valves within the atriopulmonary connection are used less frequently. Some groups have reported that venous valves used in atriopulmonary shunts contribute little to the postoperative hemodynamics and that patients fare no better than those without venous valves. These observations, along with the high incidence of implanted valve–related complications, have led most surgical teams to abandon use of venous valves.[49–53] However, this concept remains controversial, and many groups, including Fontan's, believe that the use of valved atriopulmonary connections is justified, particularly in patients with marginally elevated pulmonary resistance.[54, 55] Similarly, complications of conduit use, primarily late obstruction, have led to their avoidance except in special situations, with most atriopulmonary shunts constructed with endogenous tissue or cryopreserved homograft.[13, 51, 56, 57]

The routine use of the Glenn operation for superior vena caval pulmo-

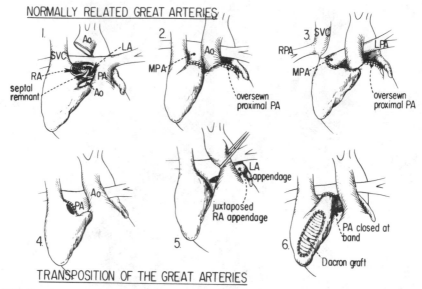

NORMALLY RELATED GREAT ARTERIES

TRANSPOSITION OF THE GREAT ARTERIES

FIG 3.
The various posterior atriopulmonary connections detailed by Doty et al. for tricuspid atresia with normally related or transposed great arteries. The atriopulmonary connection directly to the right pulmonary artery was described without detachment of the main pulmonary artery **(1)**. Detachment of the main pulmonary artery and direct anastomosis to the atrial appendage was described either alone **(2)** or in combination with a Glenn shunt **(3)**. With transposition of the great arteries, the direct atriopulmonary connection was described with the main pulmonary left in place **(4)** or with the main pulmonary artery detached and anastomosed directly to the right atrial appendage **(5 and 6)**. (From Doty DB, Marvin WJ Jr, Lauer RM: Modified Fontan procedure: Methods to achieve direct anastomosis of the right atrium to pulmonary artery. *J Thorac Cardiovasc Surg* 1981; 81:470–477. Used by permission.)

nary diversion has also become less common. Although early proponents noted that the Glenn operation may provide some protection should late obstruction develop, the decrease in conduit use and Kreutzger's findings that an atriopulmonary anastomosis provided an adequate correction obviated its benefits in most situations. In addition to the fact that it adds to the surgical complexity, a physiologic disadvantage of including the classical Glenn shunt in the Fontan procedure is that it may cause an imbalance in distribution of pulmonary blood flow by directing the lesser superior vena cava blood return to the larger right lung and the greater inferior vena cava blood flow to the smaller left lung.[58] Thus, if it has not been previously constructed, it is rarely used in combination with routine direct atriopulmonary connections.[50, 57, 58]

The early experience with complete diversion of venous to pulmonary circulation was primarily in patients with tricuspid atresia. Modifications of

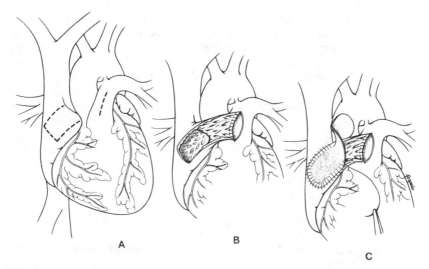

FIG 4.
Direct anterior atriopulmonary anastomosis accomplished without detachment of the pulmonary artery or insertion of a valve. A "trap door" is constructed in the right atrial appendage **(A)** and its leading edge attached to a longitudinal incision in the main pulmonary artery **(B)**. The anterior defect is closed with a pericardial patch **(C)**. (From Michler RE, Rose EA, Malm JR: Tricuspid atresia, in Arciniegas E (ed): *Pediatric Cardiac Surgery*. Chicago, Year Book Medical Publishers, 1985, p 297. Used by permission.)

the procedures were developed for application to other forms of complex univentricular heart disease, particularly, in patients with two atrioventricular valves or absent left atrioventricular valve.[57, 59] Simple or patch closure of the atrial septal defect combined with direct closure of the right-sided atrioventricular valve was used initially to separate the venous return in patients with an adequate left-sided atrioventricular valve. Alternately, to utilize the right-sided atrioventricular valve, methods of separating the venous return were developed using intra-atrial baffles, either to direct the pulmonary venous blood through the atrial septal defect and to the right atrioventricular valve, or more recently to direct the inferior vena cava blood return along the lateral aspect of the right atrium, away from the atrioventricular valve, to the roof of the atrium and superior vena cava, where the atriopulmonary shunt is then constructed.[59–61]

With improved results and wider application of the Fontan procedure,[62, 63] additional modifications have been developed that allow concomitant repair of associated lesions. Correction of associated lesions (e.g., partial or total anomalous pulmonary venous return, Ebstein's anomaly, atrioventricular canal, criss-cross heart, straddling atrioventricular valves, transposition of the great arteries, subaortic obstruction, left-sided superior or inferior vena cava, pulmonary stenosis, and pulmonary atresia) concomitant with a modified Fontan procedure has also been reported.[57–61, 64–71]

Thus in present clinical practice the term "modified Fontan procedure" has evolved to describe a wide variety of procedures that share the common goals of separating the systemic and pulmonary circulation, directing the pulmonary venous return exclusively to the functional ventricular component, and establishing a systemic to pulmonary connection that relies on increased systemic venous pressure rather than on a functional ventricle to provide adequate pulmonary blood flow and ventricular diastolic filling. These procedures, originally developed to treat tricuspid atresia, now allow complete correction of many complex forms of "univentricular" cardiac malformations that would otherwise have a poor prognosis.

Physiologic Considerations

The beneficial physiologic effects of the modified Fontan procedure include relief of cyanosis and elimination of ventricular volume overload. However, after this procedure there are basic physiologic changes that relate to the absence of a functional "pulmonary" ventricle. In these patients systemic venous pressure must be elevated to become the principal driving force to maintain both adequate pulmonary blood flow and ventricular preload. If pulmonary vascular anatomy and pulmonary vascular resistance are normal, modest and well-tolerated increases in systemic venous pressure are usually sufficient to provide adequate pulmonary blood flow; however, these patients will have less reserve capacity to deal with physiologic impedence to pulmonary blood flow or with compromise in ventricular function.[55, 58, 61, 72-74]

Increased pulmonary vascular resistance occurs frequently in patients with univentricular hearts, and these patients will require greater increases in venous pressure after modified Fontan procedures to maintain pulmonary blood flow.[58, 61, 72-75] Inappropriate early palliation may result in either excessive pulmonary blood flow, with the development of reactive or fixed pulmonary vascular disease, or conversely, insufficient pulmonary blood flow, with subsequent inadequate growth and development of the pulmonary circulation.* In addition, pulmonary artery stenosis may occur primarily or as a result of technical complications of shunt placement, and can also add to pulmonary resistance. Failure to reverse these abnormalities before or at the time of repair may lead to the requirement for excessive systemic venous pressure in the postoperative period and greater potential for low cardiac output.†

Similarly, after atriopulmonary connection, factors such as pneumothorax, pleural effusion, pericardial effusion, and positive-pressure ventilation, which reduce venous return and increase resistance to pulmonary blood flow, can severely compromise cardiac output and are poorly tolerated.[58, 74, 76]

Because systemic venous pressure must also provide adequate left ven-

*References 5, 8, 12, 13, 16, 20, 58, 60, 70.
†References 5, 8, 13, 57, 58, 70, 75.

tricular filling, compliance and systolic function are equally important physiologic considerations. A stiff, noncompliant ventricle, as might be seen with an associated outflow obstruction, may demand an elevated filling pressure to achieve adequate preload. Similarly, a poorly contractile ventricle, as might occur with excessive preoperative volume load, may also require elevated filling pressure to achieve the greater preload needed to achieve adequate stroke volume. These patients will require a greater increase in systemic venous pressure to maintain the higher filling pressure's needed to support adequate postoperative cardiac output.*

Persistent intracardiac left-to-right shunts may result from inadequate closure of a ventricular septal defect in repairs using a hypoplastic right ventricle in the systemic venous to pulmonary connection, incomplete closure of the pulmonary valve after a direct atriopulmonary connection, or incomplete closure of the tricuspid valve with repair of univentricular atrioventricular connections. Extracardiac left-to-right shunting may occur if palliative shunts or major aortopulmonary collateral arteries are not completely controlled. Postoperatively a left-to-right shunt will increase pulmonary blood flow, thereby increasing pulmonary pressure, and, in addition, will place an increased volume load on the ventricle, and thus increase the ventricular filling pressure. These changes will be reflected in higher systemic venous pressure necessary to maintain adequate systemic cardiac output.[57, 58, 73, 74, 77]

Patient tolerance of postoperative systemic venous hypertension depends primarily on the magnitude of the increase in systemic venous pressure. If the systemic venous pressure required to maintain systemic perfusion in the postoperative period remains below 17 mm Hg, sequelae are minimal. If higher systemic venous pressure is required, large volume fluid administration may be required to maintain the necessary elevation of venous pressure in the early postoperative period, and subsequent pleural and pericardial effusions as well as hepatic congestion, peripheral edema, ascites, and even protein-losing enteropathy may occur.†

The role of atrial contractions, as well as the pumping action of the small right ventricular segments included as part of the atriopulmonary connection, in augmenting pulmonary blood flow in the postoperative period is a subject of considerable controversy. Many have found that atrial contraction contributes little to improving pulmonary blood flow.‡ and may, by causing turbulence, impede pulmonary blood flow.[61] Others believe that the right atrium, particularly if hypertrophied as with tricuspid atresia, may be capable of aiding pulmonary circulation, and advocate the use of a valve within the atriopulmonary connection.[50, 52, 54, 55]

The incorporation of a hypoplastic right ventricle into the systemic venous to pulmonary connection was proposed by Bowman[47] and Bjork[48] and their co-workers to more effectively augment pulmonary blood flow,

*References 5, 12–15, 60, 65, 74, 75.
†References 54, 57, 58, 65, 74, 78.
‡References 52, 53, 58, 72, 79, 80.

with the degree of augmentation related to the size and development of the right ventricle.[81] The Toronto group[82] reported improved survival and lower postoperative right atrial pressure in repair of tricuspid atresia that included the right ventricle in the right atrium to right pulmonary artery connection. However, studies comparing pulmonary artery and systemic venous pressures have failed to show any increase as the result of incorporation of a hypoplastic right ventricle in the connection,[23] and pulmonary blood flow patterns after modified Fontan procedures appear unrelated to the presence or absence of a hypoplastic right ventricle within the repair.[72] Furthermore, significant contractions of an incorporated right ventricle may result in significant regurgitation into the atrium,[48] and insertion of a valve within the atrioventricular connection may be required.[46, 57, 58, 81]

Patient Selection

Important considerations in patient selection include the age, cardiac diagnosis, and physiologic parameters. Proper patient selection depends on the presence of cardiac anatomy amenable to repair with a modified Fontan procedure and on physiologic parameters that suggest that the patient will tolerate such repair without excessive risk for complications or death. The timing of surgery is controversial and requires consideration of the status of the patient's physiologic development, as well as the presence and nature of symptoms. The optimal age for a patient to undergo the modified Fontan operation should be individualized to allow time for adequate growth and development of the pulmonary circulation but to avoid excessive delays that may lead to compromise of ventricular function or development of pulmonary vascular disease. Proper selection of patients and timing of surgical intervention may be as critical to a successful outcome as are proper performance of the procedure and appropriate postoperative management.[58, 73, 74]

In most series, the greatest experience and best operative results have been obtained in patients with tricuspid atresia. Other forms of univentricular heart, univentricular atrioventricular connection, "massive" ventricular septal defect, straddling atrioventricular valve, and pulmonary atresia with intact ventricular septal defect with appropriate physiologic features also benefit from the modified Fontan procedure, and in recent series excellent results have been obtained in these groups.[14, 57, 60]

Patients with two atrioventricular valves may also be considered for septation as an alternative to the modified Fontan procedure. In most reports, however, mortality related to septation is high and postoperative heart block and ventricular dysfunction common.[83, 84] With the improved results reported in these patients after repair with the modified Fontan procedure, septation may best be limited to selected patients with a double-inlet left ventricle and an anterior aorta or small subaortic outlet chamber and those patients with univentricular heart who are not physiological candidates for the modified Fontan procedure.[14, 60, 83–85]

In 1977 Choussat et al.[74] proposed criteria for patient selection for Fontan repair, based on review of their early experience: (1) at least 4 years of age, (2) sinus rhythm, (3) normal caval drainage, (4) normal-sized right atrium, (5) mean pulmonary artery pressure less than or equal to 15 mm Hg, (6) pulmonary artery resistance less that 4 U/m^2, (7) pulmonary arteries equal in diameter to 75% or more of the diameter of the aorta, (8) ventricular ejection fraction of 60% or more, (9) absence of atrioventricular valve regurgitation, and (10) no impairing effects from prior shunting.

These criteria, based on the physiologic principles noted above, were designed to select patients likely to have good pulmonary and systemic perfusion without requiring excessive increase in systemic venous pressure. Although these criteria are in principle valid, advances in surgical techniques, myocardial protection, and postoperative care have vastly increased the number of patients who are suitable candidates for these repairs.[58, 63, 65, 76]

In general, candidates should have adequate circulation with a pulmonary vascular resistance less than 2 U/m^2, and a mean preoperative pulmonary artery pressure of less than 15 to 20 mm Hg. Patients with a pulmonary vascular resistance of more than 4 U/m^2 or decreased ventricular function with ejection fraction less than 45% or end-diastolic pressure of greater than 15 mm Hg are poor candidates and should be denied the procedure.

There is flexibility in each of the selection criteria. Higher pulmonary resistance may be acceptable in patients with excellent cardiac function and low ventricular filling pressure, because the resultant pulmonary artery and right atrial pressures are usually acceptable. Conversely, moderately depressed cardiac function may be acceptable if the pulmonary resistance is very low. Preoperative pulmonary pressure above 20 mm Hg may be due to excessive pulmonary blood flow, and if systemic saturation is high and calculated pulmonary vascular resistance low, these patients are usually acceptable as well. Pulmonary pressure above 25 mm Hg, even with acceptable calculated resistance, is worrisome. In these patients we usually prefer to perform a palliative procedure that includes a Glenn shunt and pulmonary artery banding to reduce pulmonary blood flow and left ventricular volume load, in anticipation of improving the pulmonary artery pressure and better preparing the patient for a later Fontan procedure.

It is recommended that the diameter of the main pulmonary artery be greater than 75% of the diameter of the ascending aorta,[74] or the ratio of the combined diameters of the left and right pulmonary arteries to the diameter of the descending thoracic aorta at the diaphragm be greater than 2.0.[13] If, however, pulmonary artery flow and pressure are good, we will operate on these patients and augment hypoplastic or stenotic pulmonary arteries as part of the modified Fontan procedure.

In general, modified Fontan procedures are avoided in patients with supraventricular arrythmias; however, in selected patients they may be well tolerated.[86] Similarly, atrioventricular valve dysfunction can be corrected as part of the procedure by valve repair or replacement.[13, 74]

The appropriate age at which a child can undergo a modified Fontan procedure is controversial. Optimal results are reported when the procedure is delayed until patients are older than 4 or 5 years, allowing complete growth, development, and maturation of the pulmonary vascular bed.* However, not all agree that it is best to delay this corrective procedure in every patient. Some patients develop or have recurrent symptoms well before this age, and further palliation after 1 year of age may result in patients becoming unsuitable candidates for a subsequent Fontan procedure.[75] In addition, the less than optimal ventricle may deteriorate before the child reaches 4 or 5 years of age, from the prolonged volume overload imposed by mixed circulation.† In these patients earlier repair may be preferred. Proponents of early repair with a modified Fontan procedure cite reports of good results in patients older than 6 to 12 months who meet the other selection criteria,[13, 62, 87] and that earlier repair reduces not only the duration that the ventricle is subjected to volume overload but also the potential negative effects of prolonged cyanosis on ventricular function and neurologic development as well as the risks for cerebrovascular embolism and brain abscess that may occur with venous mixing.[8, 13, 62, 75, 88]

A compromise is probably the best approach. Patients with cardiac lesions that will require a modified Fontan procedure should be followed closely after initial evaluation. In the first months of life, symptomatic children should undergo a palliative procedure. Beyond 6 months to 1 year, children that develop recurrent symptoms of cyanosis or evidence of early ventricular compromise should undergo an "early" modified Fontan procedure. On the other hand, patients that remain symptom-free, retain good ventricular function, demonstrate adequate growth and development of the pulmonary vasculature, and are not at risk for developing pulmonary vascular disease should be operated at an elective age, usually 4 to 5 years of age.

With this philosophy, we have accepted 157 patients for the modified Fontan procedure over the last 10 years. The approach has evolved somewhat toward accepting patients who are younger and have higher preoperative pulmonary pressures. As can be seen in Table 1 the average age varied considerably. The youngest candidate accepted was 8 months of age and 21 (13%) patients were less than 2 years of age. Conversely, 22 patients were accepted after 15 years of age with the oldest patient being 38 years of age. The various cardiac diagnoses are shown in Table 2. Tricuspid atresia was not the most common diagnosis in our series and was present in 55 patients (35%). Univentricular atrioventricular connection was the most frequent diagnosis and was present in 94 patients (60%). Seven patients had pulmonary atresia with intact ventricular septum (4.4%), and 1 patient had previously undergone palliation for hypoplastic left heart syndrome.

As shown in Table 3, 83% of patients had undergone one or more palliative procedures. Table 4 shows the preoperative hemodynamics. Mean

*References 13, 51, 57, 65, 73–75.
†References 8, 12, 14, 20, 57, 75.

TABLE 1.
Profile of Patients Undergoing the
Modified Fontan Procedure

Average age	8 yrs (8 mos–38 yrs)
Male	93
Female	64
Patients < 2 yrs	21
Patients < 5 yrs	60
Patients 5–15 yrs	75
Patients >15 yrs	22

TABLE 2.
Preoperative Diagnoses of Patients
Undergoing the Modified Fontan
Procedure

Tricuspid atresia	55(35%)
Univentricular heart	94(60%)
Pulmonary atresia with intact ventricular septum	7(4.4%)
Hypoplastic left heart syndrome	1(.6%)

TABLE 3.
Prior Palliative
Procedures (83% of
Patients)

Blalock-Taussig shunt	70
Potts	6
Waterston	10
Glenn	16
Central shunt	12
PA band	39
Collateral band	1
Damus-Stansel-Kaye	1
Total	155

TABLE 4.
Preoperative Hemodynamic Profile of Patients
Undergoing the Modified Fontan Procedure*

Mean pulmonary artery pressure	15 ± 7 mm Hg (5–30 mm Hg)
Ratio of pulmonary and systemic flow	1.5 ± 0.7
Pulmonary vascular resistance	2.0 ± 1.5 (0.2–4 wood units)
Ventricular end diastolic pressure	9 ± 3 mm Hg (3–20 mm Hg)

*Pulmonary vascular resistence less than 2 wood units is preferred. A pulmonary vascular resistence of 4 wood units, or an LVEDP of 20 mm Hg may be tolerable if other parameters are ideal.

preoperative pulmonary artery pressures were 15± 7mm Hg and mean pulmonary vascular resistances were 2.0±1.5 wood units. Average ventricular end diastolic pressures were 9±3 mm Hg. Patients with mean pulmonary arterial pressures above 20 mm Hg and compromised left ventricular function were accepted only in the presence of excessive pulmonary blood flow. Patients with elevated pulmonary vascular resistances were accepted in the presence of excellent ventricular function and usual pulmonary artery pressures.

Surgical Strategy

General Considerations of Surgical Options

Because of the vast array of congenital cardiac malformations, often occurring with other noncardiac congenital defects that are now amenable to repair with the modified Fontan procedure, it is most important that the surgeon take an individual approach to each patient. As there are many options for planning an appropriate procedure, it is helpful to review several important considerations. These include (1) the method for separation of the systemic and venous return; (2) the pathway for establishment of a direct, unobstructed connection between the systemic venous return and the pulmonary arteries; (3) whether a valve should be included in the atriopulmonary connection; (4) whether a hypoplastic right ventricle chamber should be incorporated into the atriopulmonary connection and; (5) how the repair of associated defects can be integrated into the procedure. The final surgical strategy should include options in each category that work well together, are appropriate for the lesion under consideration, and are least likely to result in later complications.

Separation of Systemic and Pulmonary Circulation

Options for separation of the venous circulation depend primarily on whether a right-sided atrioventricular valve is present, and if present whether it must be incorporated into the left-sided circulation. In patients with tricuspid atresia the right-sided atrioventricular valve is of no consideration, and separation of the venous circulation can be achieved by closure of the atrial septal defect[51, 54, 73] to isolate the pulmonary venous blood to the left atrium and the systemic venous blood to the right atrium.

In lesions with a right-sided valve, it may simply be closed to create a situation similar to tricuspid atresia,[89] or can be included in the left atrioventricular connection.[90] The former option is viable only when there is an additional, normal left-sided atrioventricular valve, and it is the preferred option if there is right atrioventricular valve regurgitation. The latter option is necessary when the left-sided atrioventricular valve is absent or dysfunctional and the right-sided atrioventricular valve component is essential for adequate, unobstructed flow of the pulmonary venous blood into the ven tricle.[57, 60, 86]

To incorporate the right atrioventricular valve into the left-sided circulation, an intra-atrial baffle must be created to isolate the pulmonary venous blood to the right atrioventricular valve and the systemic venous blood to the atriopulmonary connection. The most common such baffle is created by placing a patch in the right atrium that encompasses the orifices of the interatrial septal defect and the right atrioventricular valve and excludes the orifices of the vena cava and the majority of the right atrial cavity.[57, 60, 85, 89] This commits the majority of the right atrial cavity to the systemic venous circulation and allows a similar variety of atriopulmonary connections as described for tricuspid atresia.

After studying right atrial flow patterns, deLeval et al.[61] reported an alternate method of separating the systemic and pulmonary venous return by isolating the systemic venous return within the right atrium and committing the majority of the atrial cavity to the left sided circulation (Fig 5). This concept was based on the authors' experimental observations that as the venous return passes through the larger contracting right atrium, turbulence is created that may actually interfere with the efficiency of continued flow of the venous return to the pulmonary circulation. Construction of a uniform inferior vena cava to pulmonary conduit in combination with a modified Glenn shunt resulted in more efficient streaming of venous return into the pulmonary arteries. Clinically, this can be accomplished by placing a patch that is based on a segment of the right lateral atrial wall and encompasses the orifices of the inferior and superior vena cava. The patch should be fashioned to create a conduit of uniform diameter between the inferior and superior vena cava. The venous to pulmonary connection is then completed by division of the superior vena cava and anastomosis of both the proximal and distal ends of the vena cava to the superior and inferior aspects of distal and proximal right pulmonary artery respectively. This inferior to superior vena caval conduit or baffle thus isolates the sys-

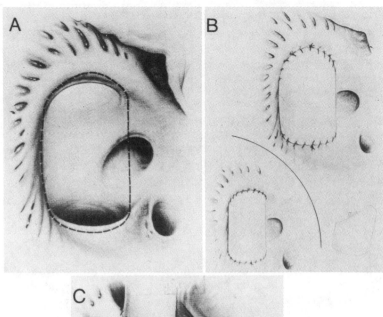

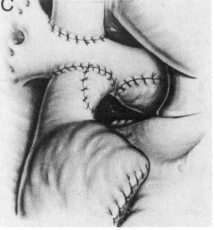

FIG 5.
The principles of the "lateral tunnel" or "cavopulmonary connection." In **A,** the dotted line shows the relationship of the intra-atrial patch to the orifices of the inferior and superior vena, the patent foramen ovale, and the coronary sinus. In **B,** the patch is shown in position. The cavopulmonary connection is shown in **C,** with direct connection of the upper and lower ends of the transected superior vena cava to the right pulmonary artery and patch augmentation of the inferior anastomosis and the proximal right pulmonary artery. (From deLeval MR, Kilner P, Gewillig M, et al: Total cavopulmonary connection: A logical alternative to atriopulmonary connection for complex Fontan operations. *J Thorac Cardiovasc Surg* 1988; 96:682. Used by permission.)

temic venous return and commits the atrial septal defect, the atrioventricular valve, the coronary sinus, and the majority of the right atrial cavity to the left sided circulation.[61]

A second consideration in achieving separation of systemic venous and pulmonary venous blood is the management of an unroofed coronary sinus or sinus septal defect with the modified Fontan operation. This condition is present in about 2% to 3% of patients with tricuspid atresia[91] but is probably more common in more complex congenital anomalies and in association with a left-sided superior vena cava. In association with modified Fontan procedures, this hard to recognize defect may not become apparent until after the repair when right atrial pressure greatly exceeds left atrial pressure and right-to-left shunting through the defect occurs. Management depends on the method of separating the venous blood. If an intra-atrial atrial septal defect to right atrioventricular valve baffle is used, extension of the patch to encompass the coronary sinus ostia, thus completely including it in the left-sided circulation, will obviate the potential problem. Similarly, the technique of isolating the caval return described by deLeval et al.[61] will also isolate the coronary sinus to the left side and eliminate potential shunting through an unroofed coronary sinus.

The danger of postoperative right-to-left shunting through an unroofed coronary sinus is greatest with tricuspid atresia or with a closed tricuspid valve when separation of venous blood is completed by closure of the atrial septal defect and the orifice of the coronary sinus is left open to the right atrium. In these situations an unroofed coronary sinus must be recognized and potential postoperative shunting prevented by direct closure of either the defect between the coronary sinus and the left atrium or the coronary sinus ostia itself.[54, 92, 93] Drainage of the coronary sinus to the left side results in minimal arterial desaturation, and because it allows drainage of the coronary veins to a lower pressure system, is preferred by many.

Systemic Venous to Pulmonary Artery Connections

Since Fontan's original procedure, modifications have evolved in the construction of the atriopulmonary connection to simplify the procedure and extend its application to other anatomic lesions. Questions as to the optimal methods of establishing a connection between the systemic venous and the pulmonary circulation, the benefits of incorporating a hypoplastic right ventricle in this connection, and whether a valve should be included have yet to be resolved. No method as yet has proved superior, and options will vary according to patient anatomy.

Kreutzer et al.[46] suggested that an inferior vena caval valve and a Glenn shunt were not necessary and demonstrated that a direct atriopulmonary connection was adequate in patients with tricuspid atresia. Advantages of the direct atriopulmonary anastomosis include its simplicity, applicability to a wide variety of malformations, and potentially lower risk for late obstruction, as reported with valved conduits. Doty et al.[56] emphasized the posterior approach, which is less susceptible to sternal compression, and summarized the possible variations of this type of connection as they might be applicable to virtually all potential variations in anatomy of the great arteries and the presence of a previous Glenn shunt. This technique has achieved excellent results in many centers and remains the most widely used in clinical practice.*

Subsequently two additional related controversies have arisen. One surrounds the potential benefits of including a hypoplastic right ventricular segment in the systemic venous connection; the other involves the use of a valve within the atrioventricular connection. Original proponents of the former suggested that a right ventricular segment incorporated into the systemic venous to pulmonary connection would add a normal endogenous valve to the circuit and, depending on contractility, may contribute to forward flow and thus improve postoperative hemodynamics.[47, 48, 81] In addition to the fact that its use is restricted to limited anatomic situations in which a hypoplastic right ventricle is indeed present, not located in the subaortic position, and not necessary for bypass of subaortic or aortic valve obstruction, potential disadvantages of the atrioventricular connection include the need for closure of a ventricular septal defect to isolate the right ventricular segment, the potential for the hypoplastic ventricle to become obstructed, and the observation that the contraction of the right ventricular segment may result in significant atrial regurgitation if an additional valve is not placed within the atrioventricular connection.†

Early benefits appear to be limited. Although the Toronto group[82] demonstrated some benefit from including the hypoplastic right ventricle in the systemic venous to pulmonary connection, in a large retrospective review of the Mayo Clinic experience atrioventricular connections fared no better than direct atriopulmonary anastomosis used with the modified Fontan procedure.[55] Similarly, Bull et al.,[81] in detailed hemodynamic studies carried out at Great Ormand Street Hospital, were unable to show improvements in the early postoperative venous to pulmonary blood flow with the incorporation of a right ventricle in left-to-right shunts in patients undergoing repair of tricuspid atresia. Pulmonary flow patterns assessed after the modified Fontan procedure show no change with the inclusion of a right ventricle in the venous circuit.[72]

Delayed hemodynamic benefits of the atrioventricular connection may occur in selected patients who demonstrate growth and improved contraction of the right ventricle years after the repair.[47, 55, 57, 81] Valve placement within the atriopulmonary connection may be necessary in these patients to achieve maximal benefits and to prevent atrial regurgitation.[47, 55, 77, 81]

Kreutzer's original procedure using a direct atriopulmonary connection included a native pulmonary valve, as noted above. However, in subsequent review of his results he found no benefit to preserving the valve in this connection and abandoned its use.[53] The majority of subsequent clinical and hemodynamic studies have shown no benefit and potential ob-

*References 13, 55, 60, 62, 71, 73, 76, 81, 85–87, 90, 94.
†References 47, 54, 55, 57, 81, 86.

TABLE 5.
Connections Used in the
Modified Fontan
Procedure*

RA to PA		112
Nonvalved	106	
Valved Conduit	6	
RA to RV		45
Nonvalved	33	
Valved conduit	12	
Glenn Shunt		28
Posterior Tunnel		2
Lateral Tunnel		12

*Nonvalved connections predominate. When a valved conduit is used, the homograft is the preferred choice.

struction with placing a valve in this connection.* One notable exception is Fontan's own studies, which consistently have shown better postoperative exercise capacity with the use of a homograft valve.[54, 73]

In our experience (Table 5), right atrial to pulmonary artery conduits were used in 112 patients (71%) while right atrial to right ventricular connections were used in 45 patients (29%). Valved connections were used in only 6 of 111 (5%) of right atrial to pulmonary artery connections and were mainly used during our early experience. Valved connections were used in 12 of 45 (27%) of right atrial to right venticular connections. Prosthetic mechanical and tissue valves were used initially; however, the availability of cyropreserved valved homograft conduits has resulted in their use in most circumstances. In addition, the lower risk of complications associated with homograft valves, and the observations that moderately developed right ventricles included in the systemic venous-pulmonary connnection could grow substantially, has lead to an increased tendency toward use of homograft valved conduits in right atrial to right ventricular connections. Classical or modified Glenn shunts were included in 28 (18%) of repairs and in conjunction with a lateral tunnel/cavopulmonary connections in 12 (8%) of patients.

Associated Anomalies

In addition to the variations in techniques for performing the modified Fontan procedure that were described above, additional modifications may be needed to deal with other associated cardiac anomalies. Atrioventricular

*References 13, 52, 57, 60, 72, 76, 79, 80, 81.

valve regurgitation may require concomitant valve repair, annuloplasty, or even valve replacement.[59, 69, 76, 85] Subaortic obstruction is also poorly tolerated and should also be corrected at the time of the modified Fontan procedure. This can be accomplished by the resection of a subvalvar membrane, the Damus-Stansel-Kaye procedure (Fig 6), the arterial switch procedure, or, if both outflow tracts are obstructive, by placement of a ventricular apical to aortic conduit.[66, 70, 71, 76, 85] Anomalous pulmonary or systemic venous return can complicate the separation of the pulmonary and systemic venous return. Adjustments of both intra-atrial baffling tech-

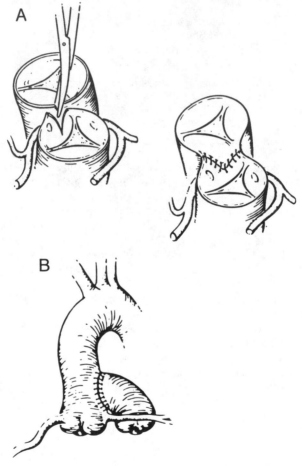

FIG 6.
Damus-Stansel-Kaye aortopulmonary anastomosis as described originally for transposition of the great arteries. The connection is begun in a side to side fashion **(A)** and completed distally by turning the end of the pulmonary artery towards the aorta **(B).** (From Mayer JE, Helgason H, Jonas RA, et al: Extending the limits for modified Fontan procedures. *J Thorac Cardiovasc Surg* 1986; 92:1021. Used by permission.)

niques and methods of atriopulmonary connection may be required to accomplish separation of the venous return (Fig 7).[76, 107, 125] In our series, anomalous pulmonary venous return was present in 6 (4%) of patients and a "posterior tunnel" was used in 2 patients to channel anomalous inferior vena caval return to the dome of the right atrium where the systemic venous to pulmonary artery connection was constructed. The Damus-

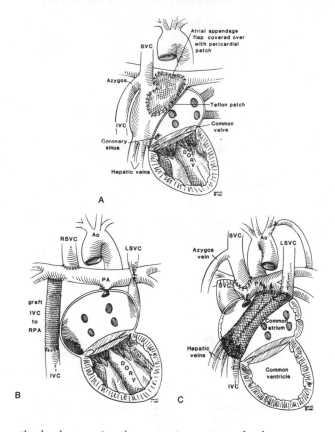

FIG 7.
Complex methods of separating the systemic venous and pulmonary venous return in patients with anomalous venous drainage. An intra-atrial baffle is modified to direct hepatic venous return with superior venacaval return to the atriopulmonary connection in a patient with azygous continuation of the inferior vena cava **(A).** Ligation of a left-sided superior vena cava and use of an extra cardiac inferior vena cava to right pulmonary artery conduit and a Glenn shunt to establish a systemic venous to pulmonary artery connection in a patient with anomalous venous drainage, common atrium, common atrioventricular valve, and double-outlet right ventricle **(B).** Use of a modified Glenn shunt and an intra-atrial conduit from the inferior vena cava and hepatic veins to a superior atrial pulmonary connection for a patient with a common ventricle, single atrioventricular connection, and left-sided superior vena cava **(C).** (From Humes RA, Feldt RH, Coburn J, et al: The modified Fontan operation for asplenia and polysplenia syndromes. *J Thorac Cardiovasc Surg* 1988; 96:212. Used by permission.)

Stansel-Kaye procedure was used in 9 (6%) of patients with obstructive lesions of the left ventricular outflow tract or aortic valve. The atrioventricular valve was repaired in 28 (18%) patients and replaced in 10 (6%) patients (Table 6).

Pulmonary Atresia With Intact Ventricular Septum

The use of the modified Fontan procedure for pulmonary atresia with an intact ventricular septum is a complicated subject and might best be considered separately. The physiologic indications for the procedure as well as the methods of achieving separation of the pulmonary venous return and atriopulmonary connection are similar to methods applicable to tricuspid atresia with an obstructed subpulmonary right ventricular chamber. The difficulties arise because of the potential deleterious effects of the hypertensive hypoplastic right ventricle and communicating right ventricular to coronary sinusoids that are frequently present when these children are evaluated for surgery. Principles for management of these problems at the time of repair are not yet elucidated, and poor results with these patients are more often caused by other factors than by complications of the modified Fontan procedure itself.

Summary of Surgical Strategies

With the diversity of lesions now considered for the modified Fontan procedure, one must be familiar with all the various surgical options that are available. Based on the above considerations we have developed a somewhat flexible approach that combines appropriate options for each individual situation with the aim of achieving maximal potential benefit while limiting unnecessary risks. In general, a direct valveless atriopulmonary connection is recommended for most candidates with good hemodynamics at preoperative evaluation. The posterior approach is preferred to avoid the potential sternal compression unless a prior Glenn shunt or other anatomic factor contraindicates this and then an anterior connection is made. A cry-

TABLE 6.
Additional Procedures Required for Adequate Repair in Patients Undergoing a Modified Fontan Procedure

Correction of partial or total anomalous pulmonary venous return	6
Damus-Stansel-Kaye procedure	9
Atrioventricular valve replacement	10
Atrioventricular valve repair	28

opreserved homograft valve may be inserted in poor hemodynamic candidates.

In patients with a subpulmonic right ventricular segment that is not obstructed and not necessary for bypass of a subaortic or aortic valve obstruction, an atrioventricular connection is used. To reduce the volume load on the hypoplastic right ventricle, a modified Glenn shunt is often constructed as part of the procedure. If the right ventricle is very hypoplastic, consisting principally of a small outflow chamber, it is not likely to develop enough function to contribute significantly to forward flow or cause troublesome regurgitation, and, therefore, no valve is included in the atrioventricular connection. If, on the other hand, the right ventricle is larger and contains some trabecular component, functional development is more likely and so a homograft valve is included in the atrioventricular connection.

Surgical Techniques

Conduct of Operation

The approach for the modified Fontan procedure is through a midline sternotomy. In young female patients with optimal anatomy and physiologic parameters, a submammary incision may be used in combination with the median sternotomy.[95] The aorta is cannulated proximal to the takeoff of the innominate artery for arterial perfusion. To allow complete atrial access, direct bicaval cannulation with right-angled metal "Pacifico" cannulas is preferred for venous drainage. Snares are placed around the superior and inferior venal caval to isolate the venous drainage, and a cardioplegia infusion cannula is placed in the proximal aorta.

Prior to commencing the repair, systemic artery to pulmonary artery shunts must be controlled. Central shunts are easily isolated on entering the chest and dissecting out the aorta and pulmonary artery. The right-sided Blalock-Taussig shunt can be approached behind the superior vena cava from its medial aspect, and the left-sided Blalock-Taussig shunt can be found by dissecting the aorta arch to the origin of the left subclavian artery.[96] Modified Blalock-Taussig shunts constructed of synthetic grafts can be approached in the same manner. Just prior to bypass these shunts should be snared down, and once bypass is accomplished, doubly ligated. Potts and Waterston shunts are occluded by compression and repaired after instituting bypass and cooling. The Waterston shunt is taken down after the aorta is cross-clamped, and the aorta repaired primarily as described for repair of tetralogy of Fallot.[97] The corresponding pulmonary artery defect can be included in an atriopulmonary connection or repaired with a patch, according to the type of systemic venous to pulmonary diversion used. Closure of a Potts shunt is carried out with deep hypothermia with low flow or circulatory arrest, carbon dioxide flooding the field, and the arch vessels occluded.[98] The aorta is closed directly, and the pulmonary artery is closed with a patch.

If a previous Glenn or modified Glenn shunt is present, direct caval cannulation and snaring of the superior vena cava above the pulmonary anastomosis provides adequate control for institution of bypass, and subsequently the shunt can be taken down or included as part of the repair.

Large aortopulmonary or bronchial collateral vessels should be closed prior to or during the modified Fontan procedure to reduce the amount of pulmonary blood flow and the volume load they impose on the ventricle. These may be closed at the time of preoperative catheterization by balloon occlusion or embolization.[99, 100] Right-sided collateral vessels may be reached by opening the anterior plural space and retracting the lung medially; left-sided collaterals may be reached by the same technique or by retracting the heart and opening the pericardium posteriorly.[101]

Once bypass has been instituted, the patient is cooled to 24°C for routine procedures, 20° to 22°C for repairs requiring periods of low flow, and even lower if periods of circulatory arrest are required. Because optimal postoperative recovery of both systolic and diastolic function is essential, meticulous techniques for myocardial protection are mandatory. We accomplish cardioplegia with cold oxygenated blood infused every 20 minutes, and additionally any time myocardial electrical activity is observed. If the patient had cyanosis prior to the repair or if the cross-clamp time is prolonged, metabolic substrates may be added, and a dose of warm substrate-enhanced blood cardioplegia may be administered prior to removal of the cross clamp.[102]

Closure of an Atrial Septal Defect

In patients with tricuspid atresia, systemic and pulmonary circulation is separated by closure of the atrial septal defect. Techniques for closure of the atrial septal defect in patients undergoing modified Fontan procedures are the same as those for closing an isolated atrial septal defect. If the edges are firm the defect can be closed primarily; however, most defects require a patch for secure closure. Because of the large pressure gradient that will occur between the two atrial chambers, secure closure is mandatory to prevent postoperative right-to-left shunting.

In patients with marginal hemodynamic status and borderline pulmonary vascular resistance, a small defect is intentionally created in the edge of the septal closure to allow a limited right-to-left shunt. The resultant "controlled" left-to-right shunt will improve the flow of blood to the left side and reduce the right atrial or systemic venous pressure necessary for adequate cardiac output while causing a level of desaturation that is acceptable.[103] Sutures are placed across the defect and brought out of the atrium near the intra-atrial groove, then passed through a snaring device. This allows narrowing or complete closure of the defect later by simply exposing the snaring device and pulling it tight.

Closure of the Tricuspid Valve

In patients with univentricular atrioventricular connection and an adequate left-sided atrioventricular valve, a situation similar to tricuspid atresia can be established by closure of the tricuspid valve. This can be particularly useful if there is tricuspid valve regurgitation. Closure of the tricuspid valve can be accomplished by direct closure of the leaflets or by suturing a patch about its orifice. Direct closure of the leaflets is usually done with interrupted, pledgetted, horizontal mattress sutures placed from the edge of one leaflet to another. Residual patency or regurgitation of the tricuspid valve can have deleterious effects, so the closure is checked carefully, and any defects are meticulously resutured. The tricuspid valve can also be closed by suturing a patch around its orifice. Care must be taken to avoid the conduction tissue that lies close to the annulus of the tricuspid valve; thus it is recommended that such a patch be sutured to the atrial wall at least 5 mm from the edge of the tricuspid annulus. In addition, if there is an unroofed coronary sinus, the patch may be placed to encompass the orifice of the coronary ostia as well.

Intra-atrial Baffles

To incorporate the right atrioventricular valve into the left-sided or systemic circulation, an intra-atrial baffle can be constructed to place the atrial septal defect in continuity with the tricuspid valve and in isolation from the vena caval orifices and systemic venous return.

Medial Atrial Septal Defect to Tricuspid Valve Baffle.—The most commonly used intra-atrial baffle used with the modified Fontan procedure involves the placement of a patch that encompasses the orifice of the atrial septal defect and the tricuspid valve.[60, 76, 85] Such a patch must be constructed so that it will not collapse in the postoperative period as the right-sided venous pressure exceeds that of the left. A large woven Dacron graft can be used to form a patch that is naturally resistant to collapse. The graft is cut to length according to the distance between the superior aspect of the atrial septal defect and the inferior aspects of the tricuspid valve and coronary sinus. The graft is then opened longitudinally from one end to the other, forming an appropriate-sized patch with a natural dome. With running sutures the patch is sewn around the superior aspect of the atrial septal defect and inferiorly to encompass the tricuspid valve and the ostia of the coronary sinus. To avoid the conduction tissue the suture line is kept 5 to 7 mm lateral to the tricuspid valve annulus.[76, 85, 124]

Lateral Tunnel or Cavopulmonary Connection.—The placement of an intra-atrial baffle to isolate the caval return, the "lateral tunnel technique" or, as described by deLeval et al.,[61] the "caval pulmonary anastomosis," is based on the concept that the most efficient continuous stream of cavopulmonary flow can be achieved by creating a uniformly sized conduit from the inferior vena cava to the pulmonary artery. Clinically, this is accomplished by placing a baffle or patch within the right atrium that isolates the inferior vena caval return along the right lateral atrial wall and directs it to the orifice of the superior vena cava as shown in Figure 5. The patch is cut to a length that is equal to the natural distance between the superior and inferior vena caval orifices and to a width equal to about two thirds of the diameter of the inferior vena cava. The inferior end of the patch is sewn around the orifice of the inferior vena cava. The anterior and posterior edges are then sewn in a superior direction to the antero-lateral and postero-lateral right atrial wall, respectively. These suture lines are continued superiorly to the anterior and posterior aspects of the superior vena cava orifice. The conduit or tunnel is completed as the upper end of the patch is sewn around the orifice of the superior vena cava. The segment of lateral right atrium included with the patch completes the wall of an intra-atrial systemic venous conduit that is only slightly greater than the inferior vena cava in diameter and thus promotes uniform flow of the inferior vena caval return to the superior vena cava. Caval pulmonary continuity is then established by transecting the superior vena cava and performing a modified Glenn shunt with the upper end of the superior vena cava, and an end to side anastomosis between the lower end of the transected superior vena cava and the more proximal right pulmonary artery. A small pericardial patch may be used to augment this latter anastomosis. By isolating the venous return along the lateral aspect of the right atrium this technique commits the intra-atrial defect, tricuspid valve, coronary sinus, as well as the majority of the right atrial cavity to the left-sided circulation.

Atriopulmonary Anastomoses

The direct atriopulmonary connection is the most commonly used method of achieving systemic venous continuity. This connection can be constructed posterior and to the right of the aorta (see Fig 3) or anterior and to the left (see Fig 4). The posterior connection is preferred because it is less vulnerable to sternal compression and obstruction. However, if the anatomy is unsuitable because of a previous Glenn shunt or a posteriorly positioned aorta in patients with normally related great arteries, the anterior connection is used.

Posterior Atriopulmonary Connection.—For the posterior approach, different variations may be required, depending on the anatomy of the great arteries.[56] In patients with transposition of the great arteries the proximal pulmonary artery is opened longitudinally on its right anterolateral aspect, and the pulmonary valve closed directly with multiple pledgetted mattress sutures. The opening in the main pulmonary artery is then extended onto the right pulmonary artery for the atriopulmonary connection. The roof of the right atrium is opened with care taken to avoid the artery to the sinoatrial node. The posterior aspect of the right atriotomy is sutured to the inferior edge of the incision in the right pulmonary artery to form the posterior wall of the atriopulmonary connection. A pericardial patch is anastomosed to the anterior aspect of the right atriotomy inferiorly and to the upper edge of the pulmonary artery incision superiorly, to complete the anterior aspect of the connection. It is important that this patch be generous so that the edges of the pulmonary artery incision are not pulled together, because this may result in partial obstruction of the connection.

If the pulmonary artery is to the left of the aorta, further mobilization of the pulmonary arteries is required. Most commonly the pulmonary artery is transected and the proximal pulmonary artery oversewn. The distal main pulmonary artery is then passed behind and to the right of the aorta, where the atriopulmonary connection is to be constructed. The atriopulmonary connection can be completed by direct anastomosis of the distal main pulmonary artery to the dome of the right atrium, or if a wider anastomosis is desired, the main pulmonary artery can be opened onto the right pulmonary artery and the connection completed as described above.

Anterior Atriopulmonary Connection.—If the great arteries are normally related and the space behind the aorta is limited, as described above, the atriopulmonary connection must be made anteriorly. This may be accomplished by two approaches. The first is begun by transecting the pulmonary artery and oversewing he proximal pulmonary artery stump. After the pulmonary artery is transected, the distal portion of the main pulmonary artery is mobilized, advanced, and rotated anteriorly to the aorta, where it is anastomosed to the right atrial appendage. If these cannot be brought together without excessive tension, a homograft or nonvalve prosthetic conduit can be interposed to complete the connection. In the other technique, the pulmonary artery is not transected. The anterior aspect of the pulmonary artery is opened longitudinally and the pulmonary valve sutured closed directly. After this, a vertical incision is made in the right atrium 1 to 2 cm medially to the edge of the right atrial appendage. Antero-medial extensions of both ends of this incision are used to form a "trap door" like flap in the anterior aspect of the right atrial appendage. This flap is advanced anteriorly to the aorta and sewn to the right side of the pulmonary arteriotomy to form the posterior wall of the connection. The right atrial to pulmonary connection is completed anteriorly by placing a generous patch of pericardium from the right lateral aspect of the atrial opening to the left side of the incision in the pulmonary artery. This patch must be generous and redundant at each end so that when the connection is filled and placed under tension the lateral edges will not be drawn together to cause an obstruction. If the right atrial appendage cannot be advanced to the pulmonary arteriotomy, a homograft or synthetic conduit can be used.

Right Atrium to Right Ventricle Connection

In patients with normally related great arteries, nonobstructed left ventricular outflow, and a subpulmonary right ventricular chamber that is unobstructed and at least as large in diameter as the pulmonary artery, a right atrioventricular connection may be preferred. A modified Glenn shunt is frequently added to this procedure to limit the volume load on the hypoplastic right ventricle, and depending on the size and contractility of the right ventricle, a valve may be included within the atrioventricular connection.

Nonvalved Right Atrioventricular Connection.—The nonvalved right atrioventricular connection is preferred when the right ventricular chamber consists of only a small, minimally contractile outflow portion. The anastomosis is performed between the right atrial appendage and an incision in the right ventricle (Fig 8). The right ventricle is opened vertically, and the ventricular septal defect is closed with a prosthetic patch. The right ventricle is then enlarged by resection of some of the trabeculae and hypertrophied muscle bands. A vertical incision is made in the atrium, similar in length to the right ventriculotomy. As described previously, the superior and inferior ends of this incision are continued anteromedially to form a trap door—like flap from the anterior right atrial appendage. After incising the trabeculations, the flap is rotated medially and anastomosed to the right edge of the ventriculotomy to form the posterior wall of the atrioven-

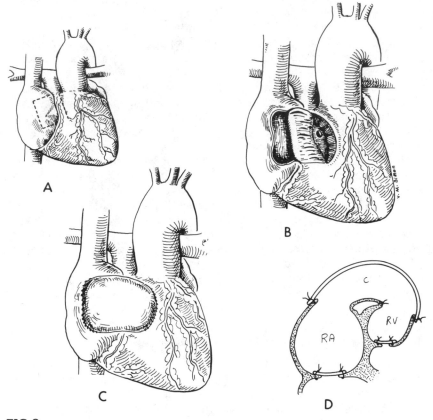

FIG 8.
Direct, nonvalved right atrial to right ventricular connection. A trap door is created in the atrial appendage and anastomosed to the right side of a longitudinal ventriculotomy **(A and B).** The anterior aspect of the connection is then completed with a pericardial patch **(C and D).** (From Laks H: Tricuspid atresia, in Glenn WWL (ed): *Thoracic and Cardiovascular Surgery,* ed 4. Norwalk, Conn, Appleton-Century-Crofts, 1983. Used by permission.)

tricular connection. The anterior wall is completed by a pericardial or synthetic patch constructed with a generous anterior bulge to avoid any potential obstruction.

Valved Right Atrioventricular Connection.—When the right ventricular chamber includes a trabecular portion and is moderate sized or contractile, a valved atrioventricular connection is preferred. As shown in Figure 9, a vertical incision is made in the right ventricle and the ventricular septal defect is closed with a patch. Large trabeculae and hypertrophied muscle bands are resected and the pulmonary valve inspected, and if questionable, calibrated. An incision is made in the right atrial appendage, and a valved homograft conduit is then used to connnect this to the right ventriculotomy. The homograft is fashioned and placed so that it will not be compressed or distorted when the heart fills and the sternum is closed.

Procedures for Associated Defects

Damus-Stansel-Kaye Operation.—In some patients undergoing the modified Fontan procedure the presence of subaortic or aortic valve obstruction may occur in the presence of unobstructed pulmonary outflow. In these cases the proximal end of the pulmonary artery can be anastomosed end-to-side to the ascending aorta, to bypass the area of obstruction, at the time of the modified Fontan procedure. As shown in Figure 6, this is ac-

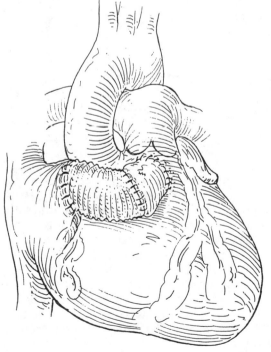

FIG 9.
Direct atrioventricular connection using a composite dacron and valved homograft conduit.

complished after the pulmonary artery has been transected to make the atriopulmonary connection. A longitudinal incision is made in the ascending aorta adjacent to the proximal pulmonary artery. A corresponding incision is made in the proximal pulmonary artery down to but not beyond the level of the valve commissures. A side-to-side anastomosis is then made between the proximal pulmonary artery and the ascending aorta until the end of the transected proximal pulmonary artery is reached. If enough proximal pulmonary artery is available, the anastomosis can be continued by suturing the end of the pulmonary artery to the remainder of the longitudinal incision in the side of the ascending aorta. Often in these patients the pulmonary arteries have been banded and there is not enough normal proximal pulmonary artery to complete such an anastomosis. In these situations, after completing the side-to-side portion of the anastomosis a pericardial or synthetic patch is used to complete the connection.[70, 104–106]

Left-Sided Modified Glenn Shunt.—In the absence of an innominate vein, the left superior vena cava should not be ligated and must be included in the systemic venous–pulmonary connection. If the left-sided superior vena cava drains into the coronary sinus, closure of a coronary sinus–left atrial communication and exclusion of the coronary ostia from the left-sided circulation, as outlined above, will suffice. If, however, a second and isolated left-sided superior vena cava drains into the left atrium, a left-sided modified Glenn shunt is used. Prior to performing this procedure the left-sided superior vena cava is clamped, and if the pressure above the clamp approaches or exceeds 20 mm hg, it is drained by insertion of a third venous cannula. The modified Glenn operation is accomplished by transecting the left-sided vena cava, closing its point of entrance into the left atrium and anastomosing it end-to-side to a longitudinal incision in the superior aspect of the left pulmonary artery.

Posterior Tunnel and Intra-atrial Conduits.—In patients with complex heterotaxia syndromes, inferior vena cava or hepatic veins draining separately into the anatomic left atrium may be isolated from the pulmonary venous return and connected with the rest of the systemic venous return by the use of intra-atrial conduits or construction of "individualized" intra-atrial tunnels (see Fig 7).[99, 107] When an intra-atrial conduit is used, one end is anastomosed to the orifice of the anomalous major vein, and the conduit is directed across the inner cavity of the atria to the dome of the atria, where the subsequent connection to the pulmonary arteries is made. Such a conduit must be positioned so that it will not obstruct the pulmonary vein or the atrioventricular valves. Tunnels, similar in principle to the cavopulmonary connection described above, can also be used to incorporate anomalous draining systemic veins. These can be created by sewing one end of a long patch around the orifice of the anomalous systemic vein and continuing the patch along the right lateral, left lateral, or even posterior aspect of the atrial cavity between the pulmonary veins. The tunnel created by this patch, like the intra-atrial conduit, is directed to an opening in the dome of the atrium, where a subsequent connection to the pulmonary circulation is constructed.

Internal Baffles for Anomalous Pulmonary Veins.—The concomitant repair of anomalous pulmonary venous return in patients undergoing the modified Fontan procedure can be accomplished successfully.[76, 99, 107] The method of repair depends on the presence or absence of a pulmonary venous confluence and eventual site of drainage into the systemic veins.[76, 99, 107–110] Total anomalous venous return to the coronary sinus is best treated by incorporation of the coronary sinus into the left-sided circulation. This can be accomplished by "unroofing" the coronary sinus into the left atrium and closing the coronary ostia, or by placing a baffle from the coronary sinus ostia to the atrial septal defect, which if necessary can include the tricuspid valve as well. With the latter approach, incision to open the coronary sinus ostia into the atrial septal defect, as described for treatment of this lesion in other circumstances, may be beneficial.[110]

Partial anomalous pulmonary venous return to the vena cava may be corrected by placement of an internal baffle to direct the pulmonary venous blood to the left side via the atrial septal defect. This is accomplished by suturing a patch within the lumen of the vena cava and the right atrium that surrounds the orifices of the anomalous pulmonary veins on one end and the atrial septal defect on the other end. When applicable, the tricuspid valve and coronary sinus may also be encompassed by the patch. The elevated systemic venous pressure that occurs following the modified Fontan procedure may tend to collapse these types of baffles and obstruct the pulmonary venous drainage, so a rigid convex patch material is used. Therefore, a rigid, convex patch material is advised. If this internal baffle causes impairment of surrounding systemic venous drainage, the vena cava may need to be enlarged with an additional patch.

Partial or total anomalous venous connection to the superior vena cava may also be treated by transection of the superior vena cava above the site of entrance of the pulmonary veins. The lower end is oversewn and the upper end anastomosed to the side of the right pulmonary artery, as in a modified Glenn operation. Total separation of the venous return may be completed by constructing a baffle to connect the orifice of the superior vena cava to the atrial septal defect, or by creating a tunnel from the orifice of the inferior vena cava to the dome of the right atrium, where a connection is established to the pulmonary arteries.

If the pulmonary veins join in the retrocardiac space, repair may be accomplished by direct anastomosis of an overlying transverse incision in the posterior wall of the left atrium to a corresponding transverse incision in the anterior aspect of the confluence of the pulmonary veins.[110] Separation of the systemic and pulmonary venous return is completed by ligation of the associated vertical vein and placement of the posterior aspect of the atrial septal defect patch or other intra-atrial baffle to the right of this anastomosis. Because of the anticipated increased right sided pressures and tendency for large right to left shunting, these latter two steps are most important in these patients.

Conclusion of the Procedure

As the cardiac repair is completed, warming is begun. A final infusion of warm blood is given, air is aspirated from the intracardiac chambers, and the cross clamp is removed. After the clamp is removed, the dome of the left atrium and the apex of the left ventricle are again aspirated for air. The cardioplegia needle is removed, leaving a small needle hole in the anterior surface of the ascending aorta to allow escape of any remaining air that is ejected from the heart. Atrial and ventricular pacing wires are inserted, and if sinus rhythm does not resume, atrial pacing is instituted. Small Silastic catheters are inserted into the right atrium, pulmonary artery, and left atrium to allow pressure monitoring in the postoperative period. After the heart is thoroughly warmed, bypass is discontinued. Most patients are weaned from bypass with only a mild dose of a pulmonary vasodilator and a cardiac inatropic agent. Volume is infused to maintain right atrial pressure increased sufficiently to support adequate pulmonary blood flow and cardiac output. In patients with marginal hemodynamic status a small externally adjustable atrial septal defect may have been created. If the right atrial pressure is less than 17 mm Hg and perfusion is good, the defect is snared closed before the operation is completed. If the required right atrial pressure is higher than 17 mm Hg the atrial communication is left open.

Prior to closing the chest, two anterior mediastinal chest tubes are placed. If either pleural space has been entered, a chest tube is placed in that pleural cavity as well. In addition, if the right atrial pressure is more than 17 mm Hg, prophylactic chest tubes may be placed in both pleural cavities, even if they previously have not been entered. As the chest is closed the position of the chest tubes as well as the atriopulmonary or atrioventricular connections are watched carefully to avoid subsequent compression and obstruction. If the right atrial pressure rises excessively with sternal closure and output decreases, the chest is immediately reopened and the cause of the problem determined. These patients tolerate tamponade very poorly, so meticulous hemostasis must be obtained prior to closing the chest.

Postoperative Management

Postoperative management is based on the physiologic principles outlined above. Emphasis is placed on the need to maintain an appropriately elevated right atrial pressure while minimizing factors that might impede pulmonary blood flow or reduce cardiac output.

In general these patients are sedated and given assisted ventilation the first night after the operation. Inatropic agents such as dopamine or dobutamine in doses of 5 μg/kg/min and pulmonary vasodilators such as nitroglycerin and nitroprusside in doses of 0.5 to 2.0 μg/kg/min are continued unless a change is indicated. Fluid is administered to maintain the right atrial pressures in the early postoperative period. However, when the peripheral vessels are fully dilated and the patient is hemodynamically stable, subsequent fluid administration is restricted and diuretics are started. Positive-pressure ventilation may have negative hemodynamic effects in these patients, so weaning and extubation are instituted as soon as the patient is awake and stable.

If the pulmonary vascular resistance and ventricular function are normal, postoperative right atrial pressure will range from 12 to 16 mm Hg. This degree of venous hypertension is usually well tolerated. Higher pressure however, is not tolerated so well and frequently results in hepatomegaly, peripheral edema, pleural effusion, pericardial effusion, and ascites. In addition, acute elevation in right atrial pressure in the early postoperative period may be associated with low-output syndrome and the need for massive fluid administration. Therefore the causes of persistently elevated or suddenly increased venous pressure must be diligently sought and corrected.

Factors that increase right atrial pressure and reduce systemic perfusion are those that impede venous return, increase pulmonary vascular resistance, and impair cardiac function. Pneumothorax, pleural effusion, pericardial effusion, and increased ventilatory pressure can have marked negative hemodynamic effects. In the face of rapid deterioration of the patient's condition, these must be investigated by appropriate studies, including careful examination of the patient, chest radiography, echocardiography, and electrocardiography. Relief of an obstructed airway or insertion of a needed chest tube may be lifesaving.

When there is hemodynamic compromise the relative changes in the right atrial, pulmonary artery, and left atrial pressure may aid in delineating the cause. A gradient between the right atrium and the pulmonary arteries suggests a mechanical obstruction in the atriopulmonary connection. Echocardiography may be helpful in confirming the presence and location of the obstruction, and these patients should be returned to the operating room for relief of the obstruction.

An increased gradient between pulmonary artery pressure and left atrial pressure is characteristic of increased pulmonary vascular resistance, common after cardiopulmonary bypass. Additional causes of increased pulmonary vascular resistance may include increased ventilatory pressure, hypercarbia, acidosis, painful stimulation, and reaction to medication or transfusion, among other endogenous factors. Measures to reduce pulmonary vascular resistance include decreasing mean airway pressure, hyperventilation, reversal of metabolic abnormalities, increased inspired oxygen concentration, sedation and relief of painful stimulation, and administration of pulmonary vasodilators. Commonly used pharmacologic pulmonary vasodilators include nitroglycerin, nitroprusside, beta adrenergic agents such as isuprel and dobutamine, alpha adrenergic blocking agents such as phentolamine, and calcium channel blockers. More recently we have found intravenously administered prostaglandin E_1 to be most effective in reducing pulmonary vascular resistance and improving perfusion, even when other agents have been ineffective. In severely elevated pulmonary vascular resistance a small controlled atrial septal defect, as described above, may dramatically improve hemodynamic status.

A primary increase in left atrial pressure with decrease in perfusion indicates depression of cardiac function. Decreased cardiac function may be confirmed by comparison of sequential echocardiograms. Therapy consists of reversal of metabolic deficits, including acidosis and hypocalcemia, administration of inatropic agents, and afterload reduction. Severely depressed cardiac function may be improved by placement of an intra-aortic balloon. We have used an IABP in 5 patients undergoing a modified Fontan, with 3 survivors.

Unfavorable hemodynamic status can also be aided by the use of a venous assist device.[111, 112] The resultant phasic lower body compression results in intermittent elevation of the venous return and right atrial pressures, resulting in increased forward flow and improved left atrial and systemic blood pressures. Fluid requirements are also reduced. We have used a venous assist device (Jobst) in 30 patients with a 70% survival rate.

In the late postoperative period, usually 6 to 8 weeks after surgery, there is a tendency for patients to develop pleural and pericardial effusions. Fluid restriction and diuretics are thus continued for at least a few months. Frequent examination, chest radiography, and echocardiography may be used to recognize these early, before hemodynamic decompensation. Although adaptation of the lymphatic vessels to compensate for the increased venous pressure does occur, frequent drainage, chest tube placement, sclerosant therapy, and even creation of a pericardial window may be required.

Results

Operative Mortality

The early reported mortality for the modified Fontan procedure was appreciable, ranging from 15% to 30% in patients with tricuspid atresia.* Subsequent improvements in patient selection, operative technique, and postoperative management have led to a significantly improved operative mortality, now reported in a number of series at 5% to 10%. The operative mortality has been significantly increased in patients with cardiac anomalies other than tricuspid atresia†; and with the improvements noted above, current series report a mortality of 10% to 20%.‡ Elevated pulmonary vascular resistance, depressed ventricular function, and atrioventricular valve dysfunction are associated with the highest mortality. The very young and the very old also are at higher risk, probably because of immature pulmonary vascular resistance in the very young patient and myocardial damage from prolonged volume overload in the older patient.

*References 13, 18, 51, 73, 76, 94, 113.
†References 13, 14, 51, 60, 76, 82, 85, 114.
‡References 14, 18, 51, 60, 62, 76, 85, 114.

TABLE 7.
Modified Fontan Procedure: Early
Mortality*

Tricuspid atresia	7.3%(4/55)
Univentricular heart	8.5%(8/94)
Pulmonary atresia with intact septum	28.6%(2/7)
Hypoplastic left heart syndrome	0%(0/1)

*Early mortality was 8.9% (14/157) for all diagnoses. Early mortality included all hospital deaths and all deaths occurring in the first 30 days following surgery.

In our experience (Table 7) there was less discrepancy in the mortality for patients with tricuspid atresia and those with univentricular atrioventricular connection. Of the 55 patients with tricuspid atresia, there were 4 early deaths (7%) while there were 8 early deaths (8%) in the 94 patients with univentricular atrioventricular connection. Patients with pulmonary atresia and intact ventricular septum comprised a smaller segment of our series (only 7 patients). Two deaths in this group resulted in a mortality rate of 29% (see Table 7).

An adjustable atrial septal defect was placed in 10 patients. Five patients were able to tolerate closure of the atrial septal defect after discontinuing bypass. The other 5 patients could not tolerate closure of the atrial septal defect as evidenced by increased right atrial pressure, decreased cardiac output and cyanosis; 3 of these were closed in the early postoperative period, and 2 remain open.

Late Mortality

Survivors of the modified Fontan procedure have an excellent prognosis. Ten-year survival of patients discharged from the hospital exceeds 90%,* and is similar regardless of the primary lesion.[85] Late mortality in our experience has occurred in 6 (4%) of 143 operative survivors (Table 8). So far there have been no late deaths of patients in our series treated for tricuspid atresia or pulmonary atresia with intact ventricular septum. There have been 6 deaths (7%) in the 86 early survivors treated for univentricular atrioventricular connection. Fontan et al.[73] reported a 14-year actuarial survival rate of more than 90%.

Late failure in early series related to conduit and valve obstruction. Presently, with the rare use of prosthetic valved conduits, late mortality appears related to arrhythmias and the development of atrioventricular valve dysfunction.[115]

*References 13, 14, 51, 60, 76, 85.

TABLE 8.
Modified Fontan Procedure: Late Mortality*

Tricuspid atresia	0%
Univentricular heart	7% (6/86)
Pulmonary atresia with intact septum	0%
Hypoplastic left heart syndrome	0%

*Late mortality was 4.2% (6/143) overall and all late deaths were confined to those patients with complex univentricular hearts.

Complications

Early complications are related to the immediate surgery and the subsequent increase in venous pressure. As noted, hepatomegaly, peripheral edema, pleural effusion, and pericardial effusion are relatively common in the first few months after surgery. Prolonged diuretic therapy and drainage of effusions is frequently required. Rarely is a pericardial window necessary. Acute liver failure[116] and systemic venous thrombosis[117, 118] have also been reported after the modified Fontan procedure.

Late complications requiring reoperation include occlusion of valves or valved conduits inserted in early repairs, atrioventricular valve regurgitation, residual atrial septal defects with right-to-left shunting, and subaortic obstruction.[115, 119] Arrhythmias,[115] cirrhosis,[120] and protein-losing enteropathy[78, 121] have also been reported as late complications related to intra-atrial suture lines, venous hypertension, and atrioventricular valve regurgitation.

In our experience (Table 9), 5 patients developed atrioventricular valve regurgitation and required valve replacement. Two patients in our early experience developed obstruction of porcine valved conduits and required replacement. Reoperations were required for closure of an unroofed coronary sinus in 1 patient, closure of residual atrial septal defects in 2 patients, resection of subaortic stenosis in 1 patient, and cardiac transplantation was required in another (see Table 9). Atrial arrhythmias requiring medication occurred in 17 (12%) patients and pacemaker implants were needed in 18 (13%) patients (Table 10).

TABLE 9.
Modified Fontan Procedure:
Reoperations*

AV valve insertion	5
Porcine conduit replacement	2
Closure unroofed coronary sinus	1
Resection subaortic stenosis	1
Cardiac transplantation	1
Closure of residual atrial septal defect	2

*Reoperation was required in 12 patients following a modified Fontan procedure. Atrioventricular valve placement for significant valvular regurgitation was the most common cause for reoperation.

TABLE 10..
Late Complications*

Significant atrial tachyarrhythmias		17
Bradyarrhythmias requiring pacemaker implantation		18
Residual Shunting		3
Unroofed coronary sinus (reop)	1	
Baffle leak	1	
Atrial septal defect (adjustable)	1	
Significant AV valve regurgitation		5
Porcine valve obstruction		2
Homograft anastomotic obstruction		1
Acquired subaortic stenosis		1

*Late complications occurring in 143 patients after a modified Fontan procedure during a mean follow-up of 40 months.

Functional Status

Functional status after modified Fontan operations is excellent, with more than 90% to 95% of patients in NYHA function class 1 or 2.[13, 73, 85, 115, 119] Nearly 90% lead normal lives and have minimal, if any, exercise restriction.[18, 51]

Hemodynamic Status

After the modified Fontan procedure, the ventricular ejection fraction is usually decreased,[88, 122] but the resting cardiac output is within normal limits.[123] In the absence of a normal subpulmonary ventricular chamber, increased cardiac output in response to exercise is achieved by an increase in right atrial pressure and in heart rate.[76, 88, 122, 123] The increase in cardiac output with exercise in these patients is limited in comparison with normal.[76, 88, 122, 123] The clinical tolerance to exercise, although less than normal, is considerable and much better than before the repair.[88, 122, 124]

Summary

The modified Fontan procedure was originated to achieve separation of the systemic and pulmonary circulation and a direct systemic venous to pulmonary connection in patients with a single functional ventricle and an otherwise poor long-term prognosis. Originally it was applied to tricuspid atresia, but subsequent modifications and improved results have extended its use to a wide variety of malformations. Controversy exists as to which modification is most advantageous, but most currently used techniques give excellent improvement in symptoms and improved short- and long-term survival.

References

1. Vlad P: Tricuspid atresia, in Keith JD, Rowe RD, Vlad P (eds): *Heart Disease in Infancy and Childhood*, ed 3. New York, Macmillan, 1978, pp 518–541.
2. Dick M, Gyler DC, Nadas AS: Tricuspid atresia: Clinical course in 101 patients. *Am J Cardiol* 1975; 36:327.
3. Rao PS: Natural history of the ventricular septal defect in tricuspid atresia and its surgical implications. *Br Heart J* 1977; 39:276.
4. Moodie DS, Ritter DG, Tajik AH, et al: Long-term follow-up of the unoperated univentricular heart. *Am J Cardiol* 1984; 53:1124.
5. Gale AW, Traill TA, Brown DJ: Abnormal ventricular function in patients with univentricular heart. *Herz* 1979; 4:226.
6. Macartney FJ, Partridge JB, Scott O, et al: Common or single ventricle: An angiocardiographic and hemodynamic study of 42 patients. *Circulation* 1976; 53:543.
7. Rahimtoola SH, Ongley DA, Swan HJC: The hemodynamics of common (or single) ventricle. *Circulation* 1966; 34:14.
8. Moodie DS, Ritter DG, Tajik AH, et al: Long-term follow-up after palliative operations for univentricular heart. *Am J Cardiol* 1984; 53:1648.
9. Blalock A, Taussig HB: The surgical treatment of malformations of the heart in which there is pulmonary stenosis or pulmonary atresia. *JAMA* 1945; 128:189.
10. Potts OWJ, Smith S, Gibson S: Anastomosis of the aorta to a pulmonary artery. *JAMA* 1946; 132:627.

11. Waterston DJ: Treatment of Fallot's tetralogy in children under one year of age. *Rozhl Chir* 1962; 41:181.
12. Taussig HB: Long-time observations on the Blalock-Taussig operation IX. Single ventricle (with apex to the left). *Johns Hopkins Med J* 1976; 139:69.
13. Kirklin JW, Barratt-Boyes BG: Tricuspid atresia, in Kirklin JW, Barratt-Boyes BG (eds): *Cardiac Surgery.* New York, John Wiley & Sons, 1986, pp 857–858.
14. Stefanelli G, Kirklin JW, Naftel DC, et al: Early and intermediate-term (10-year) results of surgery for univentricular atrioventricular connection ("single ventricle"). *Am J Cardiol* 1984; 54:811.
15. Muller WH, Damman JF: Treatment of certain congenital malformations of the heart by the creation of pulmonic stenosis to reduce pulmonary hypertension and excessive pulmonary blood flow (a preliminary report). *Surg Gynecol Obstet* 1952, 95:213.
16. Vilani M, Crupi G, Locatelli G, et al: Experience in palliative treatment of univentricular heart including tricuspid atresia. *Herz* 1979; 4:256–261.
17. LaCorte MA, Dick M, Scheer G, et al: Left ventricular function in tricuspid atresia: Angiographic analysis in 28 patients. *Circulation* 1975; 52:996.
18. Brux JL, Zannini L, Binet Jp, et al: Tricuspid atresia: Results of treatment in 115 children. *J Thorac Cardiovasc Surg* 1983; 85:440.
19. Kyger ER III, Reul GJ Jr, Sandiford FM, et al: Surgical palliation of tricuspid atresia. *Circulation* 1975; 52:685.
20. Trusler GA, Williams WG: Long-term results of shunt procedures for tricuspid atresia. *Ann Thorac Surg* 1980; 29:312.
21. Taussig HB, Keinonen R, Momberger N, et al: Long-term observations on the Blalock-Taussig operation IV: Tricuspid atresia. *Johns Hopkins Med J* 1973; 132:135.
22. Carlon CA, Mondini PG, DeMarchi R: Surgical treatment of some cardiovascular diseases (a new vascular anastomosis). *J Int Coll Surg* 1951; 16.1.
23. Glenn WWL, Patino JF: Circulatory bypass of the right heart: I. Preliminary observations on the direct delivery of vena caval blood into the pulmonary arterial circulation: Axygos vein–pulmonary artery shunt. *Yale J Biol Med* 1954; 27:147.
24. Glenn WWL: Circulatory bypass of the right side of the heart: II. Shunt between the superior vena cava and distal right pulmonary artery: Report of a clinical application. *N Engl J Med* 1958; 259:117.
25. Bakulev AN, Kolesnikov SA: Anastomosis of superior vena cava and pulmonary artery in the surgical treatment of certain congenital defects of the heart. *J Thorac Surg* 1959; 37:693.
26. Edwards JE, Bargeron LM Jr: The superiority of the Glenn operation for tricuspid atresia in infancy and childhood. *J Thorac Cardiovasc Surg* 1968; 55:60.
27. di Carlo D, Williams WG, Freedom RM, et al: The role of cava-pulmonary (Glenn) anastomosis in the palliative treatment of congenital heart disease. *J Thorac Cardiovasc Surg* 1982; 83:437.
28. Mathur M, Glenn WWL: Long-term evaluation of caval pulmonary artery anastomosis. *Surgery* 1973; 74:899.
29. Bargeron LM Jr, Karp RB, Barcia A, et al: Late deterioration of patients after superior vena cava to right pulmonary artery anastomosis. *Am J Cardiol* 1972; 30:211.
30. Laks H, Mudd JG, Standeven JW, et al: Long-term effect of the superior

vena cava–pulmonary artery anastomosis on pulmonary blood flow. *J Thorac Cardiovasc Surg* 1977; 74:253.

31. Robicsek F, Sanger PW, Moore M, et al: Observations following four years of complete circulatory exclusion of the right heart. *Ann Thorac Surg* 1969; 8:530.

32. Starr I, Jeffers WA, Meade RH: The absence of conspicuous increments of venous pressure after severe damage to the right ventricle of the dog, with a discussion of the relation between clinical congestive failure and heart disease. *Am Heart J* 1943; 26:291.

33. Robard S, Wagner D: Bypassing the right ventricle. *Proc Soc Exp Biol Med* 1949; 71:69.

34. Warden HE, DeWall RA, Varco RL: Use of the right auricle as a pump for the pulmonary circuit. *Surg Forum* 1954; 5:16.

35. Robicsek F, Temesvari A, Kadar R: A new method for the treatment of congenital heart disease associated with impaired pulmonary circulation. *Acta Med Scand* 1956; 154:151.

36. Haller JA, Adkins JC, Worthington M, et al: Experimental studies on permanent bypass of the right heart. *Surgery* 1966; 59:1128.

37. Just-Viera JO, Rive-Mora E, Altieri PI, et al: Tricuspid atresia and the hypoplastic right ventricular complex: Complete correction for long-term survival. *Surg Forum* 1971; 22:165.

38. Hurwitt EW, Young D, Escher DJW: The rationale of anastomosis of the right atrial appendage to the pulmonary artery in the treatment of tricuspid atresia. *J Thorac Surg* 1955; 30:503.

39. Shumaker HB: Discussion of Hurwitt et al. *J Thorac Surg* 1955; 30:503.

40. Harrison, 1962.

41. Fontan F, Baudet E: Surgical repair of tricuspid atresia. *Thorax* 1971; 26:240.

42. Fontan F, Mournicot FB, Baudet E, et al: Correction de latresie tricuspidienne. Rapport de deux cas "corriges" par l'utilisation d'un tecnique chir-urgical nouvelle. *Ann Chir Thorac Cardiovasc* 1971; 10:39.

43. Ross DN, Somerville J: Surgical correction of tricuspid atresia. *Lancet* 1973; 1:845.

44. Stanford W, Armstrong RG, Cline RE, et al: Right atrium–pulmonary artery allograft for correction of tricuspid atresia. *J Thorac Cardiovasc Surg* 1973; 66:105.

45. Miller RA, Pahlajani D, Serratto M, et al: Clinical studies after Fontan's operation for tricuspid atresia. *Am J Cardiol* 1974; 33:157.

46. Kreutzer G, Galíndez E, Bono H, et al: An operation for the correction of tricuspid atresia. *J Thorac Cardiovasc Surg* 1973; 66:613.

47. Bowman FO Jr, Malm JR, Hayes CJ, et al: Physiologic approach to surgery for tricuspid atresia. *Circulation* 1978; 58(suppl):83.

48. Bjork VO, Olin CL, Bjarke BB, et al: Right atrial–right ventricular anastomosis for correction of tricuspid atresia. *J Thorac Cardiovasc Surg* 1979; 77:452–458.

49. Koiwaya Y, Watanabe K, Orita Y, et al: Contrast two-dimensional echocardiography in diagnosis of tricuspid atresia. *Am Heart J* 1981; 101:507.

50. Stanton RE, Lurie PR, Lindesmith GG, et al: The Fontan procedure for tricuspid atresia. *Circulation* 1981; 64(suppl 11):140.

51. Gale AW, Danielson GK, McGoon DC, et al: Fontan procedure for tricuspid atresia. *Circulation* 1980; 62:91–96.

52. Ishikawa T, Neutze JM, Brandt PWT, et al: Hemodynamics following the

Kreutzer procedure for tricuspid atresia in patients under 2 years of age. *J Thorac Cardiovasc Surg* 1984; 88:373.

53. Kreutzer GO, Vargas FJ, Schlicht AJ, et al: Atriopulmonary anastomosis. *J Thorac Cardiovasc Surg* 1982; 83:427.
54. Ottenkamp J, Rohmer J, Quaegebeur JM, et al: Nine years' experience with physiologic repair of tricuspid atresia: Long term results and current surgical approach. *Thorax* 1982; 37:718.
55. Lee CN, Schaff HV, Danielson GK, et al: Comparison of atriopulmonary versus atrioventricular connections for modified Fontan/Kreutzer repair of tricuspid valve atresia. *J Thorac Cardiovasc Surg* 1986; 92:1038.
56. Doty DB, Marvin WJ Jr, Lauer RM: Modified Fontan procedure: Methods to achieve direct anastomosis of the right atrium to pulmonary artery. *J Thorac Cardiovasc Surg* 1981; 81:470–477.
57. Laks H, Williams WG, Hellenbrand WE, et al: Results of right atrial to right ventricular and right atrial to pulmonary artery conduits for complex congenital heart disease. *Ann Surg* 1980; 192:382.
58. Laks H: Tricuspid atresia, in Glenn WWL (ed): *Thoracic and Cardiovascular Surgery,* ed 4. Norwalk, Conn, Appleton-Century-Crofts, 1983.
59. McGoon DC, Danielson GK, Ritter DC, et al: Correction of the univentricular heart having two atrioventricular valves. *J Thorac Cardiovasc Surg* 1977; 74:218.
60. Gale AW, Danielson GK, McGoon DC, et al: Modified Fontan operation for univentricular heart and complicated congenital lesions. *J Thorac Cardiovasc Surg* 1979; 78:831.
61. deLeval MR, Kilner P, Gewillig M, et al: Total cavopulmonary connection: A logical alternative to atriopulmonary connection for complex Fontan operations. *J Thorac Cardiovasc Surg* 1988; 96:682.
62. Stellin G, Mazzucco A, Bortolotti U, et al: Tricuspid atresia versus complex lesions: Comparison of results with a modified Fontan procedure. *J Thorac Cardiovasc Surg* 1988; 96:204.
63. Marcelletti C, Mazzera E, Olthof H, et al: Fontan's operation: An expanded horizon. *J Thorac Cardiovasc Surg* 1980; 80:764.
64. Marcelletti C, Duren DR, Schuilenburg RM, et al: Fontan's operation for Ebstein's anomaly. *J Thorac Cardiovasc* 1980; 79:63.
65. Mayer JE, Helgason H, Jonas RA, et al: Extending the limits for modified Fontan procedures. *J Thorac Cardiovasc Surg* 1986; 92:1021.
66. Freedom RM, Williams WG, Fowler RS, et al: Tricuspid atresia, transposition of the great arteries, and banded pulmonary artery. Repair by arterial switch, coronary artery reimplantation and right atrioventricular valved conduit. *J Thorac Cardiovasc Surg* 1983; 85:447.
67. Uretzky G, Puga FJ, Danielson GK: Modified Fontan procedure in patients with previous ascending aorta–pulmonary artery anastomosis. *J Thorac Cardiovasc Surg* 1983; 85:447.
68. Dick M, Behrendt DM, Byrum CJ, et al: Tricuspid atresia and the Wolf-Parkinson-White syndrome: Evaluation, methodology and successful surgical treatment of the combined disorders. *Am Heart J* 1981; 101:496.
69. Jennings RB, Crisler C, Johnson DH, et al: Tricuspid atresia with dextrotransposition, dextrocardia, and mitral insufficiency: Successful circulatory correction. *Ann Thorac Surg* 1980; 29:369.
70. Waldman JD, Lamberti JJ, George L, et al: Experience with Damus procedure. *Circulation* 1988; 78:32.
71. Russo P, Danielson GK, Puga FJ, et al: Modified Fontan procedure for biven-

tricular hearts with complex forms of double-outlet right ventricle. *Circulation* 1988; 78:20.

72. DiSessa TG, Child JS, Perloff JK, et al: Systemic venous and pulmonary arterial flow patterns after Fontan's procedure for tricuspid atresia or single ventricle. *Circulation* 1984; 70:898.

73. Fontan F, Deville C, Quaegebeur J, et al: Repair of tricuspid atresia in 100 patients. *J Thorac Cardiovasc Surg* 1983; 85:647.

74. Choussat A, Fontan F, Besse P, et al: Selection criteria by Fontan's procedure, in Anederson RH, Shinebourne EA (eds): *Paediatric Cardiology*. Edinburgh, Churchill Livingstone, 1977, p 559.

75. Mietus-Snyder M, Lang P, Mayer J, et al: Childhood systemic-pulmonary shunts: Subsequent suitability for Fontan operation. *Circulation* 1987; 76:39.

76. Laks H, Milliken J, Perloff JK, et al: Experience with the Fontan procedure. *J Thorac Cardiovasc Surg* 1984; 88:939.

77. Sade R, Castaneda AR: Tricuspid atresia, in Sabiston DC, Spencer FC (eds): *Gibbon's Surgery of the Chest*. Philadelphia, WB Saunders Co, 1976, pp 1152–1169.

78. Hess J, Kruizinga K, Bijileveld CM, et al: Protein-losing enteropathy after Fontan operation. *J Thorac Cardiovasc Surg* 1984; 88:606.

79. Shemin RJ, Merrill WH, Pfeifer JS, et al: Evaluation of right atrial pulmonary conduits for tricuspid atresia. *J Thorac Cardiovasc Surg* 1979; 77:685.

80. Nakazawa M, Nakanishi T, Okuda J, et al: Dynamics of right heart flow in patients after Fontan procedure. *Circulation* 1984; 69:306.

81. Bull C, deLeval MR, Stark J, et al.: Use of a subpulmonary ventricular chamber in Fontan circulation. *J Thorac Cardiovasc Surg* 1983; 85:21.

82. Coles JG, Leung M, Kielmanowicz S, et al: Repair of tricuspid atresia: Utility of right ventricular incorporation. *Ann Thorac Surg* 1988; 45:384.

83. Feldt RH, Mair DD, Danielson GK, et al: Current status of the septation procedure for univentricular heart. *J Thorac Cardiovasc Surg* 1981; 82:93.

84. McKay R, Pacifico AD, Blackstone EH, et al: Septation of the univentricular heart with subaortic outlet chamber. *J Thorac Cardiovasc Surg* 1982; 84:77.

85. Kirklin JW, Barratt-Boyes BG: Univentricular atrioventricular connection (single ventricle), in Kirklin JW, Barratt-Boyes BG (eds): *Cardiac Surgery*. New York, John Wiley & Sons, 1986, pp 1301–1327.

86. Behrendt DM, Rosenthal L: Cardiovascular status after repair by Fontan procedure. *Ann Thorac Surg* 1980; 29:322.

87. Coles JG, Kielmanowicz S, Freedom RM, et al: Surgical experience with the modified Fontan procedure. *Circulation* 1987; 76:61.

88. del Torso S, Kelly MJ, Kalff V, et al: Radionuclide assessment of ventricular contraction at rest and during exercise following the Fontan procedure for either tricuspid atresia or single ventricule. *Am J Cardiol* 1985; 55:1127.

89. diDonato R, Becker AE, Nijveld A, et al: Ventricular exclusion during Fontan operation: An evolving technique. *Ann Thorac Surg* 1985; 39:283.

90. Ashraf H, Cotroneo J, Han S, et al: Right atrial to pulmonary artery diversion for double inlet ventricle (abstract). *J Am Coll Cardiol* 1985; 5:478.

91. Rumisek JD, Pigott JD, Weinberg PM, et al: Coronary sinus septal defect associated with tricuspid atresia. *J Thorac Cardiovasc Surg* 1986; 92:142.

92. Kurosawa H, Yagi Y, Imamura E, et al: A problem in Fontan's operation: Sinus septal defect complicating tricuspid atresia. *Heart Vessels* 1985; 1:48.

93. Quaegebeur J, Kirklin JW, Pacifico AD, et al: Surgical experience with unroofed coronary sinus. *Ann Thorac Surg* 1979; 27:418.

94. Annecchino FP, Brunelli F, Borghi A, et al: Fontan repair for tricuspid atresia: Experience with 50 consecutive patients. *Ann Thorac Surg* 1988; 45:430.
95. Laks J, Hammond GL: A cosmetically acceptable incision for the median sternotomy. *J Thorac Cardiovasc Surg* 1980; 79:146.
96. Sade RM, Bernhard WF, Castaneda AR: Ligation of subclavian to pulmonary artery shunt: Simplified technique. *Ann Thorac Surg* 1970; 17:407.
97. Ebert PA, Gay WA Jr, Oldham HM: Management of aorta–right pulmonary artery anastomosis during total correction of tetralogy of Fallot. *Surgery* 1972; 71:231.
98. Kirklin JW, Karp RB: The Tetralogy of Fallot From a Surgical Viewpoint. Philadelphia, WB Saunders, 1970, p 88.
99. Szarnicki R, Krebber HJ, Wack J: Wire coil embolization of systemic–pulmonary artery collaterals following surgical correction of pulmonary atresia. *J Thorac Cardiovasc Surg* 1981; 81:124.
100. Grinnell VS, Mehringer CM, Hieshima GB, et al: Transaortic occlusion of collaterla arteries to the lung by detachable valved balloons in a patient with tetralogy-of-Fallot. *Circulation* 1982; 65:1276.
101. Matsuda H, Hirose H, Nakano S, et al: Management of enlarged aortopulmonary collateral arteries in patients with ventricular septal defect and pulmonary atresia: Simultaneous ligation through median sternotomy during intracardiac repair. *Ann Thorac Surg* 1985; 40:593–598.
102. Rosenkranz ER, Okamoto F, Buckberg GD, et al: Safety of prolonged aortic clamping with blood cardioplegia: III. Aspartate enrichment of glutamate blood cardioplegia in energy depleted hearts after ischemic and reperfusion injury. *J Thorac Cardiovasc Surg* 1986; 91(3):428.
103. Pearl J, Laks H, Haas GS, et al: The use of an adjustable intra-atrial communication in patients undergoing the Fontan and definitive right heart procedures, submitted for publication.
104. Stansel HC: A new operation for d-loop transposition of the great vessels. *Ann Thorac Surg* 1975; 19:565.
105. Kaye MP: Anatomic correction of transposition of the great arteries. *Mayo Clin Proc* 1975; 50:638.
106. Lin AE, Laks H, Barber G, et al: Subaortic obstruction in complex congenital heart disease: Management by proximal pulmonary artery to ascending aorta end to side anastomosis. *J Am Coll Cardiol* 1986; 7:617.
107. Humes RA, Feldt RH, Coburn J, et al: The modified Fontan operation for asplenia and polysplenia syndromes. *J Thorac Cardiovasc Surg* 1988; 96:212.
108. Whight CM, Barratt-Boyes BG, Calder AL, et al: Total anomalous pulmonary venous connection. *J Thorac Cardiovasc Surg* 1978; 75:52.
109. Katz NM, Kirklin JW, Pacifico AD: Concepts and practices in surgery for total anomalous pulmonary venous connection. *Ann Thorac Surg* 1978; 25:479.
110. Kirklin JW, Barratt-Boyes BG: Total anomalous pulmonary venous connection, in Kirklin JW, Barratt-Boyes BG (eds): *Cardiac Surgery*. New York, Churchill Livingstone, 1988, p 499.
111. Heck HA, Doty DB: Assisted circulation by phasic external lower body compression. *Circulation* 1981; 64:118.
112. Milliken JC, Laks H, George B: Use of a venous assist device after repair of complex lesions of the right heart. *J Am Coll Cardiol* 1986; 8:922.
113. Cleveland DC, Kirklin JK, Naftel DC, et al: Surgical treatment of tricuspid atresia. *Ann Thorac Surg* 1984; 38:447.

114. Kirklin JK, Blackstone EH, Kirklin JW, et al: The Fontan operation: Ventricular hypertrophy, age, and date of operation as risk factors. *J Thorac Cardiovasc Surg* 1986; 92:1049.
115. Girod DA, Fontan F, Deville C, et al: Long-term results after the Fontan operation for tricuspid atresia. *Circulation* 1987; 75:605.
116. Matsuda H, Covino E, Hirose H, et al: Acute liver dysfunction after modified Fontan operation for complex cardiac lesions: Analysis of the contributing factors and its relation to an early prognosis. *J Thorac Cardiovasc Surg* 1988; 96:219.
117. Okita Y, Miki S, Kusuhara K, et al: Massive systemic venous thrombosis after Fontan operation: Report of a case. *Thorac Cardiovasc Surg* 1988; 36:234.
118. Putman JB, Lemmer JH, Rocchini AP, et al: Embolectomy for acute pulmonary artery occlusion following Fontan procedure. *Ann Thorac Surg* 1988; 45:335.
119. deVivie E-R, Rupparth G: Long-term results after the Fontan procedure and its modifications. *J Thorac Cardiovasc Surg* 1986; 91:690.
120. Lemmer JH, Ckoran AG, Behrendt DM, et al: Liver fibrosis (cardiac cirrhosis) five years after modified Fontan operation for tricuspid atresia. *J Thorac Cardiovasc Surg* 1983; 86:757.
121. Crupi G, Locatelli G, Tiraboschi R, et al: Protein-losing enteropathy after Fontan operation for tricuspid atresia (imperforate tricuspid valve). *J Thorac Cardiovasc Surg* 1980; 28:359.
122. Shacher GB, Furhman BP, Wang Y, et al: Rest and exercise hemodynamics after the Fontan procedure. *Circulation* 1982; 65:1043.
123. Peterson RJ, Franch RH, Fajman WA, et al: Noninvasive determination of exercise cardiac function following Fontan operation. *J Thorac Cardiovasc Surg* 1984; 88:263.
124. Driscoll DJ, Danielson GK, Puga FJ, et al: Exercise tolerance and cardiorespiratory response to exercise after the Fontan operation for tricuspid atresia or functional single ventricle. *J Am Coll Cardiol* 1986; 7:1087.
125. King RM, Puga FJ, Danielson GK, et al: Extended indications for the modified Fontan procedure in patients with anomalous systemic and pulmonary venous return, in Doyle EF, Engle MA, Gersony EM, et al (eds): *Pediatric Cardiology: Proceedings of the Second World Congress.* New York, Springer-Verlag, 1986, p 523.

Immunosuppression for Cardiac Transplantation

Bruce Reitz, M.D.

Johns Hopkins University, Baltimore, Maryland

When cardiac transplantation in humans was first performed in December 1967, the understanding of transplant immunosuppression was limited.[1] Protocols of drug administration followed those used for kidney transplantation. The graft had to function immediately and continuously; there was no alternative, such as dialysis for kidney transplantation, and the side effects and toxicity of immunosuppressive therapy after cardiac transplantation were prohibitive. The situation was not much different than the observation by Alexis Carrel[2] in 1914: "The surgical side of transplantation of organs is now completed as we are now able to perform transplantation of organs with perfect ease. . . All our efforts must now be directed toward the biologic methods which will prevent the reaction of the organism against foreign tissue." Understandably, enthusiasm for the procedure declined, and all but a few centers discontinued heart transplantation in the 1970s. Despite difficulties of immunosuppression, many important principles of patient selection and management were developed, endomyocardial biopsy and distant graft procurement among them. With this approach, 1-year patient survival was 60% to 70% in the most experienced centers in 1980.[3]

Although patient survival had improved, cardiac transplantation remained difficult, and it was restricted to only six centers in the United States. Then came the introduction of cyclosporine for cardiac transplantation in late 1980, and its more widespread application in 1983. This led to an explosion in the development of new cardiac transplant centers and in the number of patients receiving cardiac transplants. Now in 1989, more than 130 heart transplant centers perform an estimated 1,600 heart transplants per year in the United States.

Although cyclosporine has simplified patient management and improved survival, there are still many problems associated with immunosuppression, and it continues to be the single most important factor in achieving good long-term results. This chapter will focus on the immunosuppressive protocols for cardiac transplantation. It will review the immunology of cardiac allograft rejection and the currently available immunosuppressive drugs with their modes of action, their side effects, and their combination in protocols that have been associated with the best outcomes.

Adv Card Surg 1:155–176, 1990
© 1990, Year Book Medical Publishers, Inc.
0889-5074/90/01-155-176-$04.00

Mechanisms of Allograft Rejection

The immune response to a transplanted heart is a complex interaction of cellular and humoral mechanisms. Cell surface alloantigens are present to varying degrees within every organ and tissue. There is no evidence to suggest that the heart is any more or less antigenic than the kidney or other organs. Unless the host immune system is suppressed, these alloantigens will elicit the rejection phenomenon and lead to graft destruction.

Recognition of foreign alloantigens will initiate two types of immune response: cell-mediated responses by T lymphocytes, and humoral (or antibody)–produced responses through B lymphocytes. The mechanisms by which these responses occur are now much better understood than previously, although many features remain to be explained. The system of immune responsiveness is obviously very complex, and there are many sites at which drugs or other treatments may be used effectively. Several reviews of our present understanding of the immune system as it relates to transplantation have recently appeared.[4, 5]

Antigens are recognized by T lymphocytes only when presented to them on the surface of cells such as macrophages and monocytes. The specific immune response involves the interaction of T and B lymphocytes. The B lymphocytes can respond to free antigen but usually require help as provided by helper factors released by specifically activated T helper lymphocytes (T_H). The activity of B cells may be suppressed by T suppressor cells (Ts), which can also suppress and inhibit the proliferation of other T lymphocytes. Human helper and suppressor T cell subpopulations can be specifically measured using the OKT series of monoclonal antibodies. These antibodies are directed against differentiation antigens on the cell surface of the T cells. For example, T helper cells are OKT4 positive and T suppressor cells are OKT8 positive. Thus, the ratio of OKT4 to OKT8 may give an indication of the relative balance of the T cells that are modulating the immune response.

The host response to antigenic stimuli is the result of a delicate balance among the subgroups of lymphocytes and macrophages, as well as the activities and concentrations of their soluble products. The interrelationship between these various lymphocyte types and the mediators that they elaborate thus determines the relative presence of acceptance or rejection of the cardiac graft at any time. The strengthening of helper-cytotoxic T cells over suppressor cells accounts for the presence of acute allograft rejection. The macrophages and monocytes that gather and present foreign antigens also produce and release nonspecific soluble factors that are essential for activation of resting T cells. These substances are known as interleukin-1 (IL-1), which then stimulate T helper cells to produce a T-cell growth factor known as interleukin-2 (IL-2). The interleukins, helper and suppressor factors, and other lymphokines, together with a number of other substances produced by lymphoid and nonlymphoid cells and yet to be defined, contribute to an intricate network of immune regulation. As the immune system responds to foreign antigen, whether by cellular or humoral mechanisms, a cascade of cytotoxic events is initiated, resulting in complement activation as well as other destructive enzyme system activation leading to phagocytosis, chemotaxis, and general disruption of cellular integrity. These complex events remain to be completely described; until then, we still do not have a good understanding of the way in which the immune response leads to graft destruction.

In contrast to the development of delayed cellular immune responses characteristic of most organ transplants, preformed antibody against antigens in common with a specific donor may exist within the recipient that will trigger an immediate immune response of greatly increased severity. This occurs in patients exposed to previous organ transplants, sensitized by previous blood transfusions, or exposed to donors of a different blood type, or in patients when exposed to organs from discordant species as in xenotransplantation. Presensitization by antibody in cardiac transplant recipients can be assessed by means of testing the recipient's serum against a panel of random donor leukocytes and assessing the degree of reactivity. The preformed reactive antibody titer is often expressed as a percentage, reflecting the number of positive interactions among a random panel of 30 to 50 individuals. The preformed reactive antibody titer is often quite high in the case of kidney transplant recipients exposed to multiple transfusions or previous transplants but is generally low or absent in cardiac transplant recipients. This can occasionally be a problem, however, particularly in patients who have had previous cardiac surgery or have previously received a cardiac transplant. In practice, then, when preformed antibody of 5% or greater is identified, a specific crossmatch between the intended donor and recipient should probably be undertaken to help prevent the possibility of an immediate or hyperacute rejection.

Mechanisms of Immunosuppression

Immunosuppressive drugs or treatments can fall into several large categories depending on the general mechanism of their action. The first approaches to immunosuppression included agents that provide a general suppression by inhibiting all rapidly dividing cells or having multiple sites of action in the scheme of immunoresponsiveness. Examples of these drugs or agents are corticosteroids, azathioprine, or whole-body irradiation.

The second type of immunosuppression is more selective, directed against T-lymphocytes, which mediate the response. Antilymphocyte globulin (ALG) or antithymocyte globulin (ATG) and monoclonal antibodies of mouse origin directed against T-lymphocyte cell surface markers (OKT3) are examples. The more selective total lymphoid irradiation (TLI) is another example.

Finally, cyclosporine is a novel type of agent that is not cytotoxic but acts by interfacing with lymphokines. It therefore is even more selective in its mode of action and disrupts communication between cells of the immune response.

Adrenal Corticosteroids

Adrenal corticosteroids are the most commonly used drugs for immuno-suppression in clinical practice and are used in a wide variety of autoim-mune illnesses as well as for the prevention and treatment of allograft re-jection. Even now, their action is incompletely understood.[6] Corticoster-oids are known to be lympholytic in certain animal species, but in man, their effects on lymphoid cell interactions is not as clear. Very high doses of corticosteroids may cause transient lymphopenia owing to a redistribution of both B and T lymphocytes from the blood into the bone marrow. Mea-surement of immunoglobulin levels shows that long-term administration of steroids will cause a reduction. Apart from these effects, corticosteroids have a dramatic influence on lymphoid cell infiltration and myocytolysis. Perhaps its major effect is the reversal of the inflammatory response initi-ated by the immune system, thus blocking cell destruction and further stimulation of the immune system. Before the use of cyclosporine, corticos-teroid administration was an essential part of both the prophylaxis of rejec-tion and the treatment of acute rejection crises. However, with the avail-ability of cyclosporine, some transplant centers employ protocols that do not include corticosteroids or that attempt to minimize their administration.

Long-term administration of corticosteroids results in a variety of adverse side effects similar to Cushing's syndrome, including peptic ulceration, aseptic necrosis of bone, weight gain, psychiatric effects, diabetes, and heightened susceptibility to infection of all types. The severity and extent of these side effects has been a major stimulus for development of alternative strategies for maintenance therapy.

Azathioprine

More than 30 years ago, it was recognized that certain drugs that were ef-fective against rapidly dividing cells could also produce immunosuppres-sion. Schwartz and Damashek[7] demonstrated that the antipurine drug 6-mercaptopurine, when administered with antigen in adult animals, could produce specific immunologic tolerance. This work led Calne[8] to examine its effectiveness in preventing renal allograft rejection. The drug acts by de-pressing DNA and RNA synthesis in lymphoid cells as a competitive inhib-itor of nucleotide synthesis. In rabbits, administration of 6-mercaptopurine may delay the onset of the secondary humoral response to bovine serum albumin or sheep red cells. In man, similar immune effects have been seen in azathioprine-treated patients after immunization with Salmonella anti-gen. The exact method of action is unclear; in conventional doses, there are no clear-cut effects demonstrable on lymphocyte subpopulations, and the drug may exert part of its effect by an anti-inflammatory activity.

Azathioprine was first used clinically for the prevention of renal trans-plant rejection in Boston in 1960.[9] Soon thereafter, the drug was com-bined with corticosteroids, which became the basic combination for trans-plant immunosuppression. Reemtsma et al.[10, 11] were the first investigators to achieve prolonged survival of cardiac allografts by using methotrexate and then azathioprine in dog cardiac transplant recipients. Subsequently, other investigators showed that immunosuppression of dog heart grafts with a combination of azathioprine and prednisone could result in prolonged survival.[12] With the first clinical cardiac transplant performed by Barnard in 1967, the combination of azathioprine and corticosteroids became the preferred method of preventing cardiac allograft rejection.

Irradiation

Whole-body irradiation in the form of x-rays was probably the earliest agent demonstrated to suppress immunity. Lymphocytes are very sensitive to radiation, as are stem cells within the bone marrow. Unfortunately, this leads to the severe toxicity associated with irradiation, which also includes gastrointestinal and cerebral cell damage.

To reduce toxicity, and to maintain maximal benefit, TLI is currently used for special circumstances. Total lymphoid irradiation is a standard treatment for Hodgkin's disease and for other lymphomas. After TLI, there is a prolonged depression of a variety of immunologic parameters, including decreased T-cell counts, lower or absent delayed hypersensitivity to intradermal antigen, and decreased reactivity of peripheral blood lymphocytes to allogeneic stimulation.[13] The immunosuppressive properties of TLI were first shown by Slavin et al.[14] in rodents. Total lymphoid irradiation has been successfully used in recipients of second or third kidney grafts and has allowed discontinuing use of steroids.[15]

Antilymphocyte or Antithymocyte Preparations

The concept of using antibodies directed against lymphocytes to depress the immune response was developed experimentally by Woodruff and Anderson.[16] Lymphocytes, or other lymphoid cells, from the species in whom immunosuppression is anticipated, are injected repeatedly into an animal of a different species. This serum, when carefully adsorbed against platelets and cells other than lymphocytes, will result in a purified preparation of gamma globulin with the desired effectiveness. Both serum and purified gamma globulin have been demonstrated to be immunosuppressive, but globulin preparations are generally less toxic. These preparations result in significant immunosuppression by initiating direct destruction or inactivation of the target cell. They are among the most potent inhibitors of cell-mediated immunity currently available. Small amounts of antilymphocyte globulin administered to mice will prolong skin grafts to four or five times their usual survival. Larger doses allow the prolonged survival of even xenografted skin.

Antilymphocyte or antithymocyte preparations have been produced in a number of animal species, and recently, by a very sophisticated monoclonal antibody technique, very purified antibody has been produced against specific subsets of lymphocytes. An example of this latter preparation is the currently available mouse antibody produced against OKT3 cells.[17] It is an IgG2a murine antibody, directed to the CD3 (T3) antigen, which is found on all T lymphocytes. By binding to the CD3 receptor, OKT3 makes the cell incapable of responding to a foreign antigen.

These agents have the additional benefit of direct measurement of their ability to depress the circulating T-cell count and to impair T-cell activity. Furthermore, titers of antibody directed against the antithymocyte, antilymphocyte, or mouse antibody of OKT3 can be separately measured to detect sensitization against the preparation itself. All of these agents have been shown to be effective as prophylaxis of rejection, particularly in the immediate posttransplant period, as well as in the treatment of acute rejection crises.

Cyclosporine

Much of the present enthusiasm for cardiac transplantation can be directly linked to the benefits derived from immunosuppression induced by cyclosporine. The relatively more specific mechanism of action of this drug confers a number of advantages over previous therapy.

Cyclosporine was initially discovered by Borel[18] as part of a screening process for the discovery of new antibiotics or antifungal agents. As part of the screening procedure, Borel tested these new drugs in a model that would detect immunosuppressive properties. While testing a fungal byproduct from a soil sample, Borel noticed relatively poor antibiotic potential, some antiprotozoal effect, but a remarkable effectiveness in a mixed lymphocyte culture assay. Borel was persistent in further elucidating the mechanism of action of this compound, and it was subsequently tested by Kostakis et al.[19] in Cambridge, England, in a rat heterotopic heart transplant model. These studies demonstrated surprisingly good graft survival, and it was subsequently tested in other animal species.[20] The compound proved to be remarkably effective in preventing allograft rejection for a variety of organs and species. This led to an initial clinical trial by Calne and coworkers[21] in renal transplantation, and then Starzl et al.[22] in hepatic transplantation and Oyer et al.[23] in cardiac transplantation. The results of these early studies demonstrated that cyclosporine was remarkably effective in its immunosuppressive properties.

Mechanisms of Action

As an immunosuppressive agent, cyclosporine is a unique compound.[24] It is a lipophilic and hydrophobic cyclic endecapeptide of which several amino acids are N-methylated. The immunosuppressive effect occurs at an early stage following exposure to the foreign antigens. It appears to inhibit the response of lymphocytes to various mitogens by blocking the response of resting T cells to IL-2. It has not been particularly effective when IL-2 stimulation of already activated T cells is initiated. Cyclosporine does not inhibit the activation of suppressor cells, however, which is a further mechanism that allows for transplant acceptance. In some systems, cyclosporine seems to inhibit the production or release of IL-2 from activated helper cells as well, thereby impeding the amplification response to an allogenic stimulus. Cyclosporine affects the humoral system as well, mostly by inhibiting the response to T-dependent antigens. However, it has no direct action on B cells or on macrophages and other accessory cells.

Thus, cyclosporine suppresses the response to new antigenic stimuli but is relatively ineffective in suppressing the response of the host to previously sensitized, specific alloantigens. It will not prevent antibody-mediated early or hyperacute rejection, and importantly, the immunosuppressive effect is not clinically long-lived. Patients removed from cyclosporine immunosuppression do not develop specific tolerance, as discontinuation of the drug is followed relatively soon thereafter by the occurrence of acute rejection.

Cyclosporine Pharmacokinetics

Cyclosporine is lipid soluble and can be administered as an oral solution or parenterally. As an oral agent, it is dissolved in ethanol and olive oil, and when used intravenously (IV), it is administered in polyoxyethylated castor oil and alcohol, which is subsequently diluted in normal saline. Because of the possibility of leeching toxic compounds from commercial plastic bags, the IV administration should always be given in glass bottles. Intramuscular administration of cyclosporine is slow and unreliable and is therefore not advocated. The oral to IV equivalent of cyclosporine is 3:1. The advantage of IV cyclosporine is the avoidance of altered absorption, which may occur in the early postoperative phase following transplantation. Bolus administration of the IV drug is not recommended because of the extremely high drug levels that follow this form of administration. Continuous drip over 24 hours with a blood level in the therapeutic range will minimize toxicity. A steady-state level is reached by 2 hours.[25]

With oral administration, peak blood levels are achieved about 3½ hours after the dose is given. The absolute bioavailability of the drug is 30% to 50% of the dose. Tissue concentration reaches a peak at about 4 to 8 hours after a single oral dose, with the highest concentration noted in the liver, pancreas, and fatty tissue. Intermediate levels are found in the heart, lung, kidney, and brain. Muscle and spinal cord have the lowest levels.[26]

Metabolism occurs predominantly in the liver, in which the cytochrome P-450 system seems to be the primary mechanism of degradation. Thus, drugs that induce or compete for the cytochrome P-450 system influence the blood or serum level of cyclosporine (Table 1). Drugs that induce cytochrome P-450 activity and thereby accelerate cyclosporine elimination include rifampin, phenytoin, and phenobarbital. Drugs that compete for cytochrome P-450 activity, thereby resulting in a decreased elimination of cyclosporine, include ketoconazole, furosemide in high doses, and erythromycin. Since the breakdown of prednisone makes use of the same cytochrome P-450 system, high doses of corticosteroids lead to a prolonged half-life of cyclosporine. Conversely, cyclosporine itself reduces prednisone clearance.

TABLE 1.
Cyclosporine Interactions With Drugs Frequently Used in Cardiac Transplant Patients

Accelerated cyclosporine elimination	Rifampin
	Phenytoin
	Phenobarbital
Decreased cyclosporine elimination	Ketoconazole
	Erythromycin
	Furosemide in high doses
Increased nephrotoxic reaction	Amphotericin B
	Gentamicin
	Melphalan
	Trimethoprin
	Cimetidine
	Acyclovir
	Indomethacin

The half-life of cyclosporine has been demonstrated to be in the range of 7 to 9 hours. The clearance of cyclosporine has been found to range from 12 to 15 ml/min/kg. Cyclosporine clearance varies with age. Children have a 40% higher drug clearance than adults and thus require more frequent administration and higher doses.[27] Pediatric heart transplant recipients should receive cyclosporine on a three times a day basis, with a total dose of between 15 and 35 mg/kg, depending on cyclosporine levels. Adults over the age of 45 require less cyclosporine because of a 30% decrease in the drug clearance. Cyclosporine drug clearance can also be altered by changes in hepatic function. Since the liver is the primary source for cyclosporine metabolism and excretion, elevations of bilirubin of greater than 2 mg/dl can cause a reduction in drug clearance requiring a reduction in cyclosporine dose. Ninety percent of cyclosporine is metabolized in the liver, and less than 10% is eliminated through the kidney.

Cyclosporine Level Measurement/Drug Monitoring

There are two methods currently used for measuring cyclosporine concentration. A radioimmunoassay (RIA) performed by a kit distributed by Sandoz detects both the parent compound and a group of cyclosporine-related metabolites. To obtain uniform results, several important variables need to be controlled, including temperature and timing of sample storage, separation and transport, and the method and frequency of measurement of the standard curve. Although much of the early clinical work used plasma or serum utilizing the RIA assay, it is recommended that whole blood be used. This obviates the variable of temperature, since temperature affects the percentage of drug that is present in red blood cells or in plasma. At

37°C, the plasma concentration is 100%, but at 21°C, the plasma concentration is closer to 30%.

High-performance liquid chromatography (HPLC) is able to differentiate the parent compound from its metabolites. The technique uses whole blood and is more time-consuming and technically difficult than the RIA assay. However, if a clinical laboratory is experienced with the technique, reliable results can be obtained. The trend has been toward establishing HPLC tests in hospital clinical laboratories and providing the service on a daily basis. This leads to more uniform results, which have an acceptably low variation, and improves patient monitoring.

The optimal drug concentration of cyclosporine is only partially understood. Most groups believe that these concentrations should be higher in the immediate posttransplant period and lower after chronic immunosuppression has been established. Since there is a great deal of variable information in the literature, depending on the type of assay and the type of blood fraction being measured, there can be a great deal of confusion in reporting drug levels. Table 2 summarizes the therapeutic ranges observed in various clinical studies based on the RIA and HPLC assays. Therapeutic levels in the posttransplant period are higher for the RIA assay on whole blood, with trough of 300 to 800 ng/ml considered therapeutic and generally nontoxic. For RIA assay on serum, the targeted levels are between 200 and 400 ng/ml, and with HPLC assay of whole blood, the targets levels are 150 to 300 ng/ml early postoperatively. At 3 and 6 months postoperatively, targeted levels are approximately 50% of these levels. In addition to cyclosporine levels, careful measurements of renal and hepatic function are also essential to monitor therapy.

Complications of Cyclosporine Therapy

Cyclosporine is associated with a number of complications, which are summarized in Table 3. Hepatotoxic and nephrotoxic reactions, abnormal hair

---

TABLE 2.
Therapeutic Ranges of Cyclosporine in Heart Transplant Recipients*

Assay/Blood Fraction	Trough Levels, ng/ml		
	Immediate	3 mo	6 mo
RIA/serum	200–400	75–150	50–150
RIA/whole blood	300–800	200–600	150–400
HPLC/whole blood	150–400	. . .	75–150

*RIA = radioimmunoassay; HPLC = high-performance liquid chromatography.

TABLE 3.
Complications of Cyclosporine Administration*

Complication	Pathogenesis	Diagnosis	Treatment
Nephrotoxic reaction	↓ renal blood flow and GFR	↑ BUN, ↑ creatinine, hyperkalemia, hyperchloremic acidosis	↓ dosage of cyclosporine
Hepatotoxic reaction	Unclear, centrilobular fatty change	↑ SGPT, ↑ SGOT, ↑ bilirubin	↓ dosage of cyclosporine
Neoplasms	Overimmunosuppression when combined with other agents	Usually B-cell lymphoma	↓ dosage of cyclosporine
Hypertension	Nephrotoxic reaction, renin release (?)	Mild to moderate elevated BP	↓ dosage of cyclosporine, conventional antihypertensive medications
Neurologic	Unknown, potentiated by hypomagnesemia	Hand tremors, seizures	↓ dosage of cyclosporine
Hypertrichosis	Unknown, exacerbated by concomitant use of minoxidil	Excessive hair growth in preexisting hair growth areas	↓ dosage of cyclosporine
Gingival hyperplasia	Unclear	Develops slowly over several months	Good oral hygiene, ↓ dosage of cyclosporine

*GFR = glomerular filtration rate; BUN = blood urea nitrogen; SGPT = serum glutamic-pyruvic transaminase; SGOT = serum glutamic-oxaloacetic transaminase; BP = blood pressure.

growth, neuropsychiatric disorders, and gum hyperplasia all seem to be dose related or reversible. Cyclosporine was initially thought to be responsible for an increased risk of lymphoma, but this has subsequently not proved to be true.[28] In the early clinical reports in renal transplants, cyclosporine in high doses was given with prednisone and azathioprine in conventional doses. The patients were thus overly immunosuppressed.

Cyclosporine is probably also important in increasing the risk of infection, although most infectious complications are less when cyclosporine is included than with the previous methods of conventional immunosuppression.[29] Although most groups are reporting a lower incidence of infection and a lower infection-related mortality with cyclosporine, it is still very important that meticulous surveillance be maintained. Fortunately, even rather severe infectious complications can be cured while continuing maintenance immunosuppression.

The most clinically significant effects of cyclosporine involve the kidneys. Almost all patient groups receiving cyclosporine have a fall in creatinine clearance, increased serum creatinine level, fluid retention, edema, and hypertension.[30] Pathologic changes have been described in the proximal convoluted tubule and also in the distal tubules, consisting of vacuolization, epithelial swelling, hydropic degeneration, and necrosis. There is increasing clinical and experimental evidence that cyclosporine produces a derangement in the prostaglandin system in the renal tubules. Indomethacin exacerbates renal dysfunction after cyclosporine administration. Cyclosporine may act by increasing urinary thromboxane B_2 level in a dose-dependent fashion, with local vasoconstriction, platelet aggregation, and release of platelet-produced thromboxane. This may explain the development of hypertension, renal ischemia, and dysfunction that is seen clinically.

In cardiac transplant recipients, there is frequently postoperative oliguria, a seemingly synergistic effect of cyclosporine and the perioperative decrease in renal output seen after cardiopulmonary bypass and major operations. Many transplant groups have adopted an alternative immunosuppressive protocol early after surgery that minimizes cyclosporine dosages. Preoperative doses of cyclosporine are usually reduced or eliminated. McGiffin and colleagues[31] modified cyclosporine administration owing to a 22% incidence of acute renal failure after transplant. They reduced cyclosporine to 0.5 to 1 mg/kg/day and gradually increased the dose based on cyclosporine levels. Rabbit ATG was given daily until therapeutic cyclosporine levels were attained. This approach markedly reduced early renal dysfunction. Others have modified the perioperative use of cyclosporine to minimize early renal toxic reaction.[32-41] A representative list of transplant centers with the preoperative cyclosporine regimen is given in Table 4.

Renal dysfunction late after cardiac transplantation results in elevated serum creatinine, which has been almost universally described. An occa-

TABLE 4.
Preoperative Immunosuppression for Heart Transplant Patients According to Institution

Institution	Cyclosporine, mg/kg
University of Alabama[31]	0.5–1.0
University of Arizona[32]	None
Cleveland Clinic[33]	None
Harefield Hospital[34]	2–10
Johns Hopkins Hospital[35]	6–10
LaPitie Hospital[36]	None
Medical College of Virginia[37]	6–10
University of Minnesota and Washington University, Missouri[38]	6–12
University of Pittsburgh[39]	None
Stanford University[40]	10–12
Texas Heart Institute[41]	2–3

sional patient will have severe renal dysfunction and require hemodialysis or even renal transplantation as a result of cyclosporine toxicity. This was the reason for late conversion of cyclosporine-treated patients to conventional immunosuppressives, as described by Hunt et al.[42]

Hepatotoxic reaction is usually seen with an increased bilirubin level and also by increases in liver enzyme levels. There are no characteristic cellular pathologic changes except for centrilobular fatty changes within the liver. There may be both biliary canalicular dysfunction and hepatocellular dysfunction. The hepatotoxic reaction associated with cyclosporine is dose dependent and reverts to normal after the dose of cyclosporine is lowered. In general, cyclosporine hepatotoxic reaction is uncommon after cardiac transplantation, and no long-term sequelae of cyclosporine hepatotoxic reaction have yet been reported.

Neurotoxic reaction is most apparent by the development of fine tremors, paresthesias, and seizures. Most of these events are dose related and resolve with discontinuance or lowering of the drug. Convulsions have been observed in some series and are not associated with focal lesions on computed tomography, abnormal spinal fluid findings, or spinal fluid pressures.[43] The electroencephalogram generally shows diffuse changes consistent with metabolic abnormalities. When anticonvulsant drugs are instituted, cyclosporine levels should be carefully monitored because of the changes that diphenyl-hydantoin or phenobarbital can induce.

Other unusual side effects include the development of hirsutism or hypertrichosis, observed in almost all patients receiving cyclosporine. These changes can be especially troublesome in female patients because of rather marked changes in body appearance and may result in psychological problems. These changes tend to regress as the dosage of cyclosporine is lowered.

Similarly, gingival hyperplasia has been observed with no particular morbidity. The combination of cyclosporine and nifedipine has resulted in an increased rate of gingival hyperplasia (51%) when compared with cyclosporine alone (8%).[44]

An increased incidence of pericardial effusion has also been reported in cyclosporine-treated patients. In the Medical College of Virginia, Richmond, prospective randomized study, six of 14 cyclosporine-treated patients experienced pericardial effusion postoperatively, whereas none of the patients on conventional therapy developed a pericardial effusion.[45] This may be related to the changes in renal function that contribute to fluid accumulation. In our experience at Johns Hopkins Hospital, Baltimore, we have not documented this incidence of pericardial effusion, and it is unclear why this has been so frequently reported in some series.

Clinical Immunosuppression

Numerous clinical protocols have been devised addressing the role of cyclosporine and other agents in the preoperative and perioperative management of heart transplant patients. The efficacy of any one protocol over others is difficult to determine. There is a lack of large randomized prospective trials of immunosuppression, although several important attempts have been made. Studies have been reported by the Medical College of Virginia[46] and by the group at Papworth in Cambridge, England.[47] Other reports have included historical controls or have analyzed sequentially treated groups of patients. Some uniformity in comparing groups of patients from different centers can be attained by a standardized method of reporting the incidence and severity of rejection, the incidence and severity of infectious complications, and the incidence and severity of other side effects of immunosuppressive therapy.

In an attempt to illustrate current practice, we will review representative protocols from major institutions involved in heart transplantation. The advantages and disadvantages of each protocol will be described, as well as the current expectation for patient survival.

Cyclosporine and Prednisone

The initial protocols for cyclosporine's use in cardiac transplantation were developed by researchers at Stanford University (Calif.) in 1980[23] and by the University of Pittsburgh in the early part of 1981.[48] Drawing on previous laboratory experience and initial results from clinical trials in renal transplantation, the protocols depended primarily on cyclosporine in combination with prednisone. In the Stanford protocol, the cyclosporine and prednisone were combined with an early course of rabbit ATG, and in the Pittsburgh protocols, cyclosporine was combined only with low-dose prednisone. Rejection episodes were treated by pulses of 1 gm of methylprednisolone on a daily basis for 3 days.

With these protocols, early survival rates, length of hospital stay, and overall freedom from major infectious complications were improved compared with previous experience. However, in the Stanford experience, there were four lymphomas within the first 28 patients, and a relatively high incidence of renal toxic reaction, manifested by hypertension and a rising serum creatinine level. In the Pittsburgh series, with relatively less immunosuppression, there was good early survival at 1 year of 80% but a significant ongoing incidence of chronic rejection that resulted in the early development of coronary artery disease and death due to chronic rejection at 1 and 2 years. Both of these experiences suggested that the relatively high doses of cyclosporine that was required, particularly early after operation, was manifested in an inordinate amount of renal toxic reaction. Occasionally even dialysis was necessary during the first 10 days to 2 weeks following transplantation.

These early protocols established the lack of sensitivity of the electrocardiogram in monitoring rejection under cyclosporine treatment and helped develop the correlation among serum cyclosporine trough levels using RIA, therapeutic efficacy, and relation to renal function.

In the second phase of cyclosporine trials at the University of Pittsburgh, the importance of using ATG for rescue therapy of rejection episodes was developed.[49] They noticed an improvement in survival by using rabbit ATG for rescue therapy following a course of pulsed doses of steroids that were ineffective. This resulted in a marked decrease in the late development of chronic rejection, and the survival at 3½ years increased to 70% with this addition to the protocol.

Cyclosporine and Azathioprine

Because of undesirable side effects of long-term oral steroids, Yacoub and associates[34] in September 1982 initiated an immunosuppressive program of cyclosporine and azathioprine as the only two agents. Their initial report demonstrated the efficacy of this protocol, and they demonstrated an 82% 1-year survival rate. Cyclosporine was administered to maintain whole blood levels of between 500 and 1,000 ng/ml (RIA) for the first month, with trough levels being maintained at a lower level of between 150 and 300 ng/ml thereafter. Azathioprine was administered to maintain a white blood cell count of greater than 4,000/mm^3.

Using this immunosuppressive regimen, 90% of patients remained steroid free at the end of 1 year. At the end of 4 years, this number was smaller, but still there were 75% of patients who were free of maintenance steroids.

The advantage of this regimen were obvious in terms of steroid sparing, although hypertension was still seen in 60% of patients. Another advantage of this protocol was the ability to perform a transplant in patients who were insulin-dependent diabetics and in patients with a history of peptic ulcer disease, or in both older and younger patient groups.

The advantages of steroid-sparing protocols was also demonstrated by the Medical College of Virginia transplant group.[37]

Cyclosporine, Prednisone, and Azathioprine

In 1983, Bolman and associates[38] at the University of Minnesota, Minneapolis, reported a series of 17 patients undergoing heart transplantation with a triple-drug immunosuppressive protocol consisting of cyclosporine, prednisone, and azathioprine. Previously, the combination of these three drugs was thought to lead to excessive immunosuppression, based on the early renal transplant trial of Calne and his colleagues[21] at Cambridge. However, by initiating cyclosporine and the other agents at lower doses, the University of Minnesota group demonstrated that patients had improved renal function, a lower incidence of rejection, and better actuarial survival of up to 88% at 1 year and 83% at 2 years. This protocol seemed to combine the efficacious properties of cyclosporine with a reduction in its side effects, particularly in terms of renal toxic reaction. It also allowed relatively more steroid sparing and reduced the need for pulsed doses of steroid or ATG, with many patients remaining free of acute rejection.

As this protocol was adopted by a larger number of transplant centers, others confirmed the relative benefits of multidrug therapies that tended to reduce the toxicity of individual drugs. When patients in the International

Heart Transplant Registry were compared depending on their immunosuppression, those with triple-drug combinations had an improved survival over those receiving cyclosporine and prednisone alone.[50] Part of this effect might be due to the fact that patients treated with three drugs tended to be transplanted after 1984 and were compared with patients transplanted between 1981 and 1983, but most centers that have had experience with both protocols have adopted triple-drug therapy as being superior. Currently, the majority of patients are receiving cyclosporine, prednisone, and azathioprine concomitantly.

The immunosuppressive protocol currently used at the Johns Hopkins Hospital is representative of triple-drug protocols. Patients are prepared preoperatively by receiving 10 mg/kg of cyclosporine orally before going to the operating room. This dose is modulated depending on the preoperative creatinine level; patients with a creatinine level of between 1.5 and 2 mg/dl receive half of the preoperative dose, and patients with a creatinine level over 2 mg/dl receive one quarter of this dose, or it is omitted. Following the completion of the procedure, 500 mg of methylprednisolone is given IV after the patient comes off of cardiopulmonary bypass. Intravenous methylprednisolone therapy is continued for a further 24 hours by administering 125 mg IV every 8 hours for three doses.

Postoperatively, cyclosporine administration is begun at a rate of 10 mg/kg/day given orally in two divided doses. The dose of cyclosporine is varied depending on the whole blood HPLC level, maintaining trough levels between 150 and 300 ng/ml. Oral prednisone is begun at 1 mg/kg/day in two divided doses and is gradually tapered to 0.4 mg/kg by 2 weeks following transplantation. It is continued at this level for 3 months and is then tapered to 0.2 mg/kg/day. Azathioprine is administered at 2 mg/kg/day depending on the white blood cell count, maintaining counts of greater than 4,000/mm³.

With this protocol, the Johns Hopkins team has achieved 93% 1-year survival. Among these patients, the incidence of rejection was 0.44 episodes per patient-month in the first 3 months, and 0.08 episodes per patient-month after 3 months. Sixty-nine percent of patients require treatment for hypertension, and 58% have some elevation of serum creatinine at 1 year after transplant. Quality of life and return to activities has been good, similar to results achieved at other centers.

Early Prophylactic Immunosuppression Using OKT3

An innovation in early induction of immunosuppression has been adopted by the Utah transplantation program under the direction of Bristow.[51] They devised a therapy that incorporated the principle of reducing corticosteroid therapy, with aggressive early prophylaxis to avoid the need for bolus corticosteroid therapy, to decrease the risk of infection or other complications in the early posttransplant period. They established a prospective randomized trial that compared OKT3 with ATG-based prophylactic protocols. These agents were combined with cyclosporine at 3 mg/kg IV preoperatively, and continued at 6 mg/kg/day orally to maintain trough serum

RIA levels of 150 to 250 ng/ml. Standard doses of methylprednisolone perioperatively were combined with 0.2 mg/kg of prednisone begun at day 1 and continued until discontinuation of the antibody-based early prophylaxis, after which prednisone was increased to 1 mg/kg/day for 7 days and then tapered and discontinued over an additional 2 weeks. Azathioprine was administered at 4 mg/kg IV preoperatively and then approximately 2 mg/kg/day postoperatively to maintain a white blood cell count between 4,000 and 6,000/mm^3. Thus, over the long term, patients would continue to take cyclosporine and azathioprine, and prednisone would not be given routinely unless required by subsequent rejection experience. These two protocols had slightly differing rates of administration of cyclosporine, different total amounts of corticosteroid, and varying durations of the lymphocytotoxic therapy and thus were not a direct randomization between ATG and OKT3. Both protocols resulted in excellent patient survival of 96% at 6 months, with a greater percentage of the OKT3-treated patients being steroid free (88%) compared with the ATG-treated patients (46%). There was also a reduction in the number of rejection episodes per patient and the number of days until the first rejection episode, both of which were more favorable in the OKT3 protocol. Because of difficulties in maintaining a supply of the ATG (horse origin, ATGAM), the Utah group settled on the OKT3 early prophylactic protocol and have continued it since that time. Their favorable results have encouraged other centers to adopt similar aggressive prophylactic protocols that include OKT3 antibody, for both heart and heart-lung transplants.

Another side arm of the Utah randomized protocol included the use of vincristine, a lymphoblastocidal agent. This drug was given after discontinuation of the ATG or OKT3 and seemed to have, as its main effect, a greater number of patients being weaned from corticosteroid maintenance. This effect was less apparent in those patients receiving the longer course of OKT3.[52]

The Utah group concluded that the OKT3-based protocols prevented rejection for the duration of administration and thus eliminated the need for augmented immunosuppression in the early posttransplant period. Furthermore, it eliminated the need for long-term steroid therapy in a majority of patients. Disadvantages of this protocol were the amounts of systemic reaction to OKT3, which included fever and headache, diarrhea and nausea, hypotension requiring vasopressors, and a small but significant incidence of noncardiogenic pulmonary edema and serum sickness. Another disadvantage is the development of antibodies to the mouse protein, which ultimately limits repeated use of OKT3. However, experience shows that patients can be successfully treated at least twice before truly important sensitization occurs.

Treatment of Acute Rejection

Rejection of the cardiac allograft is most frequently determined by the endomyocardial biopsy. There is some variability in the interpretation of biopsies and some confusion with early ischemic changes within the first 2 weeks after transplant.[53] Thus, rejection frequency will vary from center to center, even when the same immunosuppressive protocol is used.

Moderate acute rejection consists of an interstitial mononuclear cell infiltrate, with some perivascular infiltrate. There are a variable number of focal areas of myocyte necrosis. Where these changes are detected, most centers will treat with augmented immunosuppression and perform a follow-up biopsy in 2 weeks, or as indicated.

The majority of transplant centers continue to use pulses of methylprednisolone for treatment of acute rejection, occurring within the first 60 days after transplantation. Later rejection can usually be treated by increases in oral prednisone with gradual taper. In our experience, late acute rejections can be reversed more easily in patients who experienced less rejection in the early posttransplant period. Table 5 gives the percentage of patients successfully treated with increased oral prednisone.

The use of ATGAM, rabbit ATG, or OKT3 monoclonal antibody, for acute rejection, constitutes rescue therapy after unsuccessful use of prednisone or methylprednisolone. Unfortunately, the availability of commercial preparations of ATGAM are currently limited, and it is not available for most patients. Similarly, rabbit ATG preparations are limited in availability, usually requiring special local arrangements for preparation. The use of OKT3 has increased markedly, and it is now the most commonly used preparation for rescue therapy. The doses of administration of these agents are given in Table 6.

Sensitization occurs frequently, especially after two or three courses. Another limitation of ATG therapy is the development of "rebound rejection." Early return of rejection after clearing of the endomyocardial biopsy may occur frequently. The incidence of this type of rejection after discontinuing OKT3 has been 63% in our experience, and was 50% after treatment with rabbit ATG, as shown in Table 7.

TABLE 5.
Acute Rejection Treatment With Oral Prednisone in 99 Patients (1983–1988)

	No. (%) of Patients	Rejections After 3 mo Successfully Treated With Oral Prednisone (%)
Rejection within the first 3 mo	82 (83)	74/153 (48)*
No rejection within the first 3 mo	17 (17)	13/21 (62)

*P < .05.

TABLE 6.
Rejection Protocols

Usual Indication	Agent	Dosage
Early moderate rejection in some patients, late moderate rejection	Oral prednisone	100 mg/day for 3 days followed by taper of 5 mg/day until baseline reached
Early moderate or severe rejection, late moderate rejection	IV methylprednisolone	1 gm/day for 3 days followed by prednisone taper
Early severe rejection, rescue therapy	ATGAM	15 mg/kg/day to reduce T-cell count to $<25/mm^3$ for 10 days
	OKT3	5 mg/kg/day to reduce T-cell count to $<25/mm^3$ for 10–14 days
	Rabbit ATG	5–10 mg/kg/day to reduce T-cell count to $<25/mm^3$ for 10–14 days

Alternative strategies for the treatment of early or persistent rejection episodes have recently been developed. Frazier and colleagues at the University of Texas (Houston), first advocated the use of increasing doses of IV cyclosporine for treatment of rejection.[54] In a series of 27 episodes of moderate rejection, patients received 1 to 3 mg/kg/day of augmented cyclosporine intravenously while continuing to take oral cyclosporine. This augmented dose of cyclosporine was given for 10 to 14 days, and the rejection was reversed 80% of the time. Cyclosporine levels increased from a

TABLE 7.
Rescue Therapy for Cardiac Allograft Rejection at the Johns Hopkins Hospital (1985–1988)

	OKT3	Rabbit ATG
No. of patients treated	21	12
Improved	16 (76%)	10 (83%)
No improvement	5	2
Rebound rejection after improvement	10 (63%)	5 (50%)

mean of 187 to 413 ng/ml during the period of increased cyclosporine, with no major side effects during this short-term use.

Similarly, Kobashigawa et al.[55] treated patients with mild acute rejection with increases in oral cyclosporine, treating 40 episodes in 28 patients. Patients were randomized to continue maintenance therapy or to have cyclosporine doses increased. The dose was increased by 50% to 100%, increasing mean trough levels from 169 to 413 ng/ml. In those patients with an actual increase in serum levels, 90% of them had no progression of rejection or a clearing of rejection, whereas 37% of those who had no increase in cyclosporine level went on to moderate acute rejection requiring further treatment.

Recently, Hunt and associates[56] from Stanford have reported the use of TLI for treatment of intractable cardiac allograft rejection. In three patients who were unresponsive to multiple courses of conventional therapy including high-dose steroids, ATG, and OKT3, serial administration of TLI was successful in promptly resolving rejection. Radiation doses ranged from 240 to 640 rads, the amount determined by the absolute T-lymphocyte count. The only side effect was mild and transient neutropenia, and patients were rejection free from 2 to 20 months after TLI. This is a promising modality for patients experiencing repeated rejection despite early and aggressive treatment with conventional agents.

Conclusion

Considerable advances have been made in immunosuppressive protocols since the introduction of cyclosporine. Although this agent has been of considerable help in improving patient survival and decreasing morbidity, there remains considerable need for improvement. The use of multiple immunosuppressive drugs in combination has been helpful, and the use of OKT3 and other monoclonal antibody preparations appears promising. The immunosuppressive properties of TLI may be useful for treatment of refractory rejection and may also play a role in the prophylaxis and induction of early immunosuppression. Finally, new immunosuppressive drugs are under development that will combine some of the immunoselectivity of cyclosporine without its side effects. Perhaps then even the sequelae of chronic rejection, particularly the development of coronary artery disease, may be prevented. For the future, protocols are necessary that induce complete immune tolerance to the cardiac allograft. This ultimate goal of transplantation will ensure the benefits of cardiac transplantation to patients dying prematurely of cardiac disease.

References

1. Barnard CN: Human cardiac transplant: An interim report of a successful operation performed at Groote Schuur Hospital. *S Afr Med J* 1967; 41:1271–1274.

2. Carrel A, quoted by Cosimi AB: Transplantation. *Bull Am Coll Surg* 1989; 74:41–47.
3. Pennock JL, Oyer PE, Reitz BA, et al: Cardiac transplantation in perspective for the future: Survival, complications, rehabilitation and cost. *J Thorac Cardiovasc Surg* 1982; 83:168–177.
4. Lafferty, Prowse SJ, Babcock S, et al: The allograft response. *Surg Clin North Am* 1986; 66:1231–1253.
5. Nossal GJV: The basic components of the immune system. *N Engl J Med* 1987; 316:1320–1325.
6. Flye MW: Immunosuppressive therapy, in Flye MW (ed): *Principles of Organ Transplantation*. Philadelphia, WB Saunders Co, 1989, pp 155–175.
7. Schwartz R, Damashek W: Drug induced tolerance. *Nature* 1959; 183:1682.
8. Calne RY: The rejection of renal homografts: Inhibitions in dogs by 6-mercapto-purine. *Lancet* 1960; 1:417.
9. Murray JE, Merrill JP, Harrison JH, et al: Prolonged survival of human kidney homografts by immunosuppressive drug therapy. *N Engl J Med* 1963; 268:1315.
10. Reemtsma K, Williamson WE Jr, Iglesias F, et al: Studies in homologous canine heart transplantation: Prolongation of survival with a folic acid antagonist. *Surgery* 1962; 52:127.
11. Reemtsma K, McCracken BH, Schlegel JA, et al: Reversal of early graft rejection after renal heterotopic transplantation in man. *JAMA* 1964; 187:691.
12. Lower RR, Dong E Jr, Shumway NE, et al: Suppression of rejection crises in the cardiac homograft. *Ann Thorac Surg* 1965; 1:645.
13. Fukz V, Strober S, Babrove A: Long-term effects of radiation on T and B lymphocytes in peripheral blood in patients with Hodgkin's disease. *J Clin Invest* 1976; 58:803.
14. Slavin SS, Reitz BA, Beiber CP, et al: Transplantation tolerance in adult rats using total lymphoid irradiation: Permanent survival of skin, heart, and marrow allograft. *J Exp Med* 1978; 174:700.
15. Najarian JS, Ferguson RM, Sutherland DER, et al: Fractionated total lymphoid irradiation as preparative immunosuppression in high risk renal transplantation. *Ann Surg* 1982; 196:442.
16. Woodruff MFA, Anderson NA: Effective lymphocyte depletion by thoracic duct fistula and administration of antilymphocyte serum on the survival of skin homografts in rats. *Nature* 1963; 200:702.
17. Cosimi AB, Colvin RB, Burton RC, et al: Use of monoclonal antibodies to T cell subsets for immunologic monitoring and treatment of recipients of renal allografts. *N Engl J Med* 1981; 305:380.
18. Borel JF: The history of cyclosporin-A and its significance, in White DJG (ed): *Cyclosporin-A: Proceedings of an International Conference on Cyclosporin-A*. New York, Elsevier North-Holland, Inc, 1982, pp 5–17.
19. Kostakis AJ, White DJG, Calne RY: Prolongation of the rat heart allograft survival by cyclosporine-A. *IRCS Med Sci* 1977; 5:280.
20. Calne RY, White DJG, Rolles K, et al: Prolonged survival of pig orthotopic heart grafts treated with cyclosporin-A. *Lancet* 1978; 1:1183–1185.
21. Calne RY, Rolles K, White DJG, et al: Cyclosporin-A initially as the only immunosuppressant in 34 recipients of cadaveric organs: Thirty-two kidneys, two pancreases, two livers. *Lancet* 1979; 2:1033.
22. Starzl TE, Klintmalm GBG, Porter KA, et al: Liver transplantation with use of cyclosporine-A and prednisone. *N Engl J Med* 1981; 305:266–269.

23. Oyer PE, Stinson EB, Reitz BA, et al: Preliminary results with cyclosporin-A in clinical cardiac transplantation, in White DJG (ed): *Cyclosporin-A: Proceedings of an International Conference on Cyclosporine-A.* New York, Elsevier North-Holland, Inc, 1982, pp 461–471.
24. VanBuren CT: Cyclosporine: Progress, problems, and perspectives. *Surg Clin North Am* 1986; 66:435–449.
25. Schroeder TJ, Myre SA, Melvin DB, et al: Efficacy and safety of constant-rate intravenous cyclosporine infusion immediately after heart transplantation. *J Heart Transplant* 1989; 8:5–10.
26. Atkinson K, Boland J, Britton K: Blood and tissue distribution of cyclosporin in humans and mice. *Transplant Proc* 1983; 15:2430–2433.
27. Kahan BD: Individualization of cyclosporine therapy using pharmacokinetic and pharmacodynamic parameters. *Transplantation* 1985; 40:457–476.
28. Penn I: Cancers following cyclosporine therapy. *Transplant Proc* 1987; 19:2211–2213.
29. Reece IJ, Painvin GA, Zeluff B, et al: Infection in cyclosporine immunosuppressed cardiac allograft recipients. *J Heart Transplant* 1984; 3:239–242.
30. Myers BD, Ross J, Newton L, et al: Cyclosporine-associated chronic nephropathy. *N Engl J Med* 1984; 311:699–705.
31. McGiffin DC, Kirklin JK, Naftel DC: Acute renal failure after heart transplantation and cyclosporine therapy. *J Heart Transplant* 1985; 4:396–399.
32. Copeland JG, Emery RW, Levinson MM, et al: Cyclosporine: An immunosuppressive panacea? *J Thorac Cardiovasc Surg* 1986; 91:26–39.
33. Stewart R, Govier A, Golding L, et al: Cardiac transplantation at the Cleveland Clinic: The first 24 months. *Cleve Clin J Med* 1988; 55:49–56.
34. Yacoub M, Alivizatos P, Khaghani A, et al: The use of cyclosporine, azathioprine, and antithymocyte globulin with or without low dose steroids for immunosuppression of cardiac transplant patients. *Transplant Proc* 1985; 17:221.
35. Baumgartner WA, Augustine S, Borkon AM, et al: Present expectations in cardiac transplantation. *Ann Thorac Surg* 1987; 43:585–590.
36. Cabrol C, Gandjbakhch I, Pavie A, et al: Heart transplantation in Paris at "La Pitie" Hospital. *J Heart Transplant* 1985; 4:476–480.
37. Katz MR, Barnhart GR, Szentpetery S, et al: Are steroids essential for successful maintenance of immunosuppression in heart transplantation? *J Heart Transplant* 1987; 6:293–297.
38. Bolman RM, Olivari MT, Saffitz J, et al: Current results with triple therapy for heart transplantation. *Transplant Proc* 1987; 19:2490.
39. Griffith BP, Hardesty RL, Trento A, et al: Five years of heart transplantation at Pittsburgh. *J Heart Transplant* 1985; 4:489–493.
40. Baldwin JC, Wolfgang TC, Shumway NE, et al: Cardiac transplantation, in Flye (MW (ed): *Principles of Organ Transplantation.* Philadelphia, WB Saunders Co, 1989, pp 385–402.
41. Macris MP, Frazier OH, VanBuren CT, et al: Improved immunosuppression for heart transplant patients using intravenous doses of cyclosporine. *Transplantation* 1989; 47:311–314.
42. Hunt SA, Stinson EB, Oyer PE, et al: Results of "immunoconversion" from cyclosporine to azathioprine in heart transplant recipients with progressive nephrotoxicity. *Transplant Proc* 1987; 19:2522.
43. Atkinson K, Biggs J, Darveniza P, et al: Cyclosporine associated central nervous system toxicity after allogeneic bone marrow transplantation. *N Engl J Med* 1984; 310:527.

44. Slavin J, Taylor J: Cyclosporine, nifedipine, and gingival hyperplasia. *Lancet* 1987; 2:739.
45. Hastillo A, Thompson JA, Lower RR, et al: Cyclosporine-induced pericardial effusion after cardiac transplantation. *Am J Cardiol* 1987; 59:1220–1222.
46. Barnhart GR, Goldman MH, Hastillo A, et al: Comparison of immunosuppression therapy following heart transplantation: Pretransfusion/azathioprine/ATG/prednisone vs cyclosporine-prednisone. *J Heart Transplant* 1985; 4:381–383.
47. Cavarocchi N, Hakim M, Cory-Pearce R, et al: A prospective randomized trial of cyclosporine and low dose prednisolone vs cyclosporine and azathioprine. *J Heart Transplant* 1985; 4:591.
48. Griffith BP, Hardesty RL, Deeb GM, et al: Cardiac transplantation with cyclosporine A and low-dose prednisone. *Ann Surg* 1982; 196:324–329.
49. Griffith BP, Hardesty RL, Bahnson HT: Powerful but limited immune suppression for cardiac transplantation with cyclosporin-A and low dose steroid. *J Thorac Cardiovasc Surg* 1984; 87:35–42.
50. Fragomeni LS, Kaye MP: The registry of the International Society for Heart Transplantation: Fifth official report, 1988. *J Heart Transplant* 1988; 7:249–253.
51. Bristow MR, Gilbert EM, Renlund DG, et al: Use of OKT3 monoclonal antibody in cardiac transplantation: Review of the initial experience. *J Heart Transplant* 1988; 7:1–11.
52. Gilbert EM, Renlund DG, O'Connell JB, et al: Immunosuppressive efficacy of vincristine in heart transplantation: A preliminary report. *J Heart Transplant* 1987; 6:369–374.
53. Billingham ME: Endomyocardial biopsy interpretation in cyclosporine treated cardiac recipients, in Emery RW, Pritzker MR (eds): *Cardiac Surgery: State of the Art Reviews*. Philadelphia, Hanley Belfus Inc, 1988, pp 641–646.
54. Colon R, Lorber MI, Frazier OH, et al: An alternative therapy for rejection in cardiac allograft recipients. *Transplant Proc, in press*.
55. Kobashigawa J, Stephenson LW, Moriguchi J, et al: Randomized study of high dose oral cyclosporine therapy for mild acute cardiac rejection. *J Heart Transplant* 1989; 8:53–58.
56. Hunt S, Strober S, Hoppe R, et al: Use of total lymphoid irradiation for therapy of intractable cardiac allograft rejection. *J Heart Transplant* 1989; 8:104.

Current Status of Temporary Circulatory Support

D. Glenn Pennington, M.D.

Department of Surgery, St. Louis University School of Medicine, St. Louis, Missouri

Marc T. Swartz, B.A.

Department of Surgery, St. Louis University School of Medicine, St. Louis, Missouri

For more than 30 years it has been possible to support the circulation at least partially by means of a mechanical device.[1, 2] Shortly after the development of cardiopulmonary bypass (CPB), attempts were made to support the circulation of patients partially with acute cardiogenic shock.[3] These early clinical trials were generally unsuccessful and were abandoned after a few years. By the mid-1960s, investigators were again ready to support patients in cardiogenic shock, and these efforts resulted in several long-term survivors.[4, 5] Over the next 5 to 6 years, development of the intra-aortic balloon pump (IABP) significantly decreased the number of candidates for ventricular assist devices (VADs),[6, 7] since the majority of patients in cardiogenic shock can be successfully treated with IABP. However, Norman et al.[8] defined a group of patients in cardiogenic shock with IABP, optimal preload levels, and maximum inotropic support who were unable to maintain the following hemodynamics: (1) cardiac index above 1.8 L/sq m/min, (2) systolic blood pressure above 90 mm Hg, (3) left and/or right atrial pressure below 20 mm Hg, (4) urine output above 20 ml/hr, and (5) systemic vascular resistance below 2,100 dynes•sec/cm[5]. When these conditions exist for more than a few hours, the chance of survival is less than 10%.[8]

These hemodynamic criteria form the basis for the selection of candidates for VADs and have become accepted as accurate predictors of nonsurvival. Several National Institutes of Health–sponsored groups began developing assist devices that could be used as VADs for periods of 1 to 2 weeks.[9–11] Subsequently, the National Heart, Lung, and Blood Institute (NHLBI) sponsored programs that included the clinical application of VADs[12] and the development of permanent implantable left ventricular assist systems (LVASs). Other groups were providing postcardiotomy circulatory support with commercially available centrifugal[13, 14] or roller pumps.[15]

Adv Card Surg 1:177–198, 1990

In the early 1980s, consistent and acceptable survival rates were obtained in patients in postcardiotomy cardiogenic shock.[16-20] While most of the experience with assist devices before 1985 was in patients after cardiotomy, patients with acute myocardial infarction (MI) shock and in the bridge-to-transplant category have attracted the attention of many groups.

There has been vigorous interest in the development and clinical use of circulatory support devices for rapid resuscitation that allow peripheral cannulation and provide partial support. These systems have the advantage of being useful in the coronary care unit or cardiac catheterization laboratory in patients who do not respond to IABP and drug therapy. If vital organ function can be maintained by devices during the initial shock period, more definitive options such as myocardial revascularization, correction of mechanical lesions, or cardiac transplantation are feasible. Commerically available centrifugal and roller pumps are being used at an increasing rate because they are readily available and inexpensive. Additionally, 2% to 10% of patients undergoing percutaneous transluminal coronary angioplasty (PTCA) are failures, of whom some develop cardiogenic shock and require immediate resuscitation.[21] Accordingly, it is expected that the number of patients requiring mechanical circulatory assistance will continue to increase over the next several years. This review describes the current status of the use of VADs, both FDA-regulated devices and commercially available pumps, and total artificial hearts (TAHs) in patients with cardiogenic shock.

Patient Selection

Protocols for patient selection are generally based on the work of Norman et al.,[8] who described hemodynamic criteria for patients with cardiogenic shock unresponsive to conventional therapy. In addition to pharmacologic support, other routine measures include the correction of arterial blood gas abnormalities, hypovolemia, cardiac arrhythmias, and hypothermia. From their data, the previously mentioned hemodynamic criteria are generally accepted as indications for mechanical circulatory support. Patients should be excluded from consideration for mechanical assistance if they have chronic renal failure, severe peripheral vascular disease, symptomatic cerebrovascular disease, cancer with metastasis, severe hepatic disease, significant blood dyscrasia, pulmonary disease associated with pulmonary arterial hypertension, or severe bacterial infections resistant to antibiotic therapy. Patients who have incurred central nervous system damage as a result of a period of inadequate perfusion before assist device insertion should also be excluded.

An important determinant of survival seems to be whether the ventricle has suffered a perioperative infarction or stunned myocardium.[22] If the latter has occurred, the chance for survival and cardiac recovery is excellent. In a group of 15 survivors of postcardiotomy cardiogenic shock treated with VADs (in the NHLBI cooperative clinical trials), 13 of 15 patients were in New York Heart Association class I or II, and half had normal or only mildly impaired ventricular function.[12] Similar data for VAD survivors of postoperative cardiogenic shock have been reported by Rose et al.[16] and Pennock et al.[17] Therefore, until more precise methods of measuring perioperative myocardial injury can be developed, patients who do not have exclusionary characteristics should be treated with VADs. Over the last several years there has been an increasing number of patients in the bridge-to-transplant category. Recent survival statistics from several bridge-to-transplant series have shown survival rates ranging from 50% to 90%.[23, 24] Small series of patients with acute MI shock treated with mechanical circulatory support are beginning to be reported.[25] However, until substantially greater numbers of patients are treated in this manner, no conclusions can be made.

VAD and Extracorporeal Membrane Oxygenation

Several approaches have been designed to allow rapid application of circulatory assistance in the intensive care unit (ICU), cardiac catheterization laboratory, or emergency room for patients with acute MI shock. The left atrial–femoral artery system (Table 1) requires transseptal puncture, so it can only be used in the cardiac catheterization laboratory.[26] Femorofemoral bypass (Fig 1) can be rapidly instituted by the percutaneous technique of Phillips[27] or by the femoral cutdown technique used by Pennington et al.[28] However, these systems will serve to provide support for only 24 to 48 hours, during which time more definitive measures should be accomplished. One such option is the insertion of a VAD before or after a cardiac operation, or as a bridge to transplantation. It is also possible to perform PTCA in some patients with acute MI shock if they are properly supported with a circulatory assist device. If cardiac repair is not possible or not planned, the question of whether to perform a thoracotomy to insert a VAD remains unanswered unless the patient is a candidate for cardiac transplantation.

The pneumatic sac–type pumps and LVASs were designed as fully integrated systems with specifically designed pumps, cannulas, and control consoles with the purpose of perfusing patients for periods of 7 to 14 days. Other systems were primarily designed for short-term (several hours) use during cardiac operations or for emergency circulatory support for a period of less than 24 hours. Several of the latter systems, including some roller pumps and centrifugal pumps, have been used successfully for several days in many patients. Contrarily, the Pierce-Donachy VAD (Fig 2) and Novacor LVAS (Fig 3) have been used without ill effects in survivors for 80 to 90 days. This suggests that the fully integrated systems are more efficient and safer. The two currently used centrifugal pumps (Fig 4; Medtronic pump is no longer available) have been used clinically with a variety of different cannulas (see Table 1), making it very difficult to determine whether fibrin or clot formation within these systems is related to the cannulas or the pumps.

The availability and cost of these devices are important determinants of

TABLE 1.
Summary of Mechanical Circulatory Assist Devices

	Investigational	Cannulation	Location	Flow Range L/min	Heparin Required	Duration
Pierce-Donachy Thoratec	Yes	Atrial, LV	Paracorporeal	4–6	Intermittent	Intermediate-long
Symbion AVAD	Yes	Atrial	Paracorporeal	4–6	Continuous	Intermediate
Symbion Jarvik-7 TAH	Yes	Replaces ventricles	Internal	5–8	Continuous	Intermediate-long
Novacor LVAS	Yes	LV	Internal	5–8	Intermittent	Intermediate-long
Thermedics LVAS	Yes	LV	Internal	5–8	Intermittent	Intermediate-long
Biomedicus	No	Atrial, Lv	Extracorporeal	4–6	Continuous	Short-intermediate
Centrimed-Sarns	No	Atrial, Lv	Extracorporeal	4–6	Continuous	Short-intermediate
Medtronic	—†	Atrial, LV	Extracorporeal	4–6	Continuous	Short
Roller Pump	No	Atriofemoral	Extracorporeal	2–4	Continuous	Short
Elecath	Yes	Atrial	Extracorporeal	4–7	Continuous	Short
Bard ECMO	No	Femorofemoral	Extracorporeal	3–5	Continuous	Short
Datascope ECMO	No	Femorofemoral (percutaneous)	Extracorporeal	3–5	Continuous	Short
Scimed ECMO	No	Femorofemoral RA-Ao	Extracorporeal	4–6	Continuous	Short

*LV = left ventricular; AVAD = atrioventricular assist device; ECMO = extracorporeal membrane oxygenation; RA = right atrial; Ao = aortic.
†No longer manufactured.

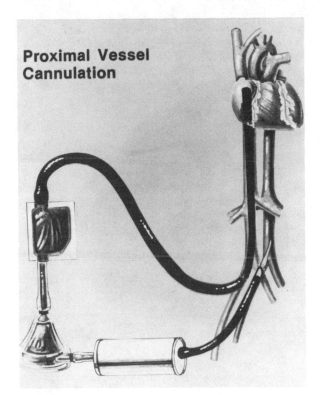

FIG 1.
Extracorporeal membrane oxygenation.

the frequency of use. Investigational VADs have been available to a limited number of institutions because of regulatory restrictions. Each manufacturer is allowed no more than 20 investigational sites per device. Since the roller and centrifugal pumps have not been restricted, many centers are using these pumps for intermediate use because of the availability and lower cost. Even with these systems, the potential use of VADs in clinical cardiac surgical practice is far from being met. Approximately 1% to 2% of all patients undergoing cardiac operations are candidates for VADs. Therefore, of the 250,000 patients undergoing cardiac operations in the United States each year, 2,500 to 5,000 are candidates. In view of these data and the increasing demand for reliable, available, and affordable devices, it is imperative that industry supply these demands. It is anticipated that every major cardiac center in the United States would like to employ some type of prolonged circulatory support system to maintain their standard of care.

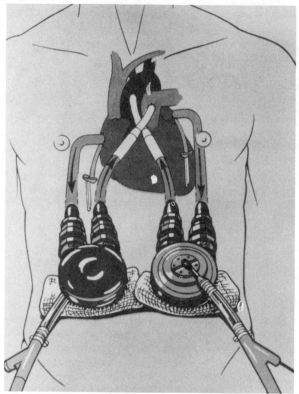

FIG 2.
The Pierce-Donachy ventricular assist device (biventricular cannulation).

Artificial Hearts

While the initial experiences with orthotopic replacement of the heart involved several different devices over the last 20 years, the most commonly used device (approximately 120 implants) is now the Symbion Jarvik-7 TAH (J-7 TAH; Fig 5). The Liotta, Akutsu, and Phoenix hearts have been used in 1 patient each, while the Pennsylvania State University Heart has been used in 2 patients; the Berlin heart and the Unger Ellipsoid heart have each been used in 4 patients. The first 2 clinical implants with a TAH in humans were done in 1969 and 1981 at the Texas Heart Institute.[29] Both of the cases were performed as bridges to cardiac transplantation. These patients subsequently underwent cardiac transplantation and died within 1 week of transplantation of sepsis and multiorgan failure. Permanent implantation of the J-7 TAH took place between 1982 and 1985. During this period, 4 patients in the United States received TAHs as permanent devices. The TAH functioned well in these patients and was able to provide adequate circulatory support, but there were frequent complica-

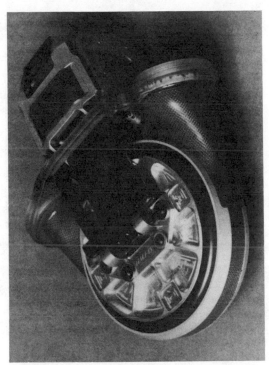

FIG 3.
Novacor left ventricular assist system (unencapsulated).

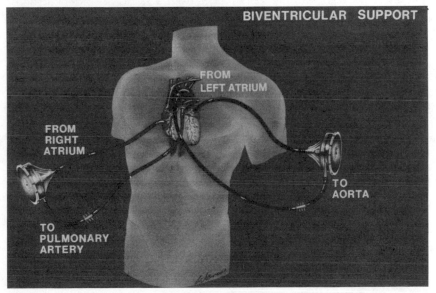

FIG 4.
Biventricular support using centrifugal pumps (Biomedicus).

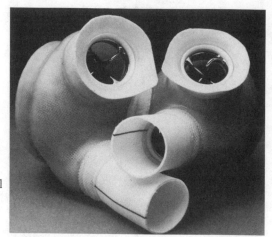

FIG 5.
Symbion Jarvik-7 total artificial heart.

tions with infection and cerebrovascular accidents (CVAs).[30, 31] While some of these neurologic events can be explained by reasons other than cerebral emboli, it is of interest that similar events have not occurred in patients who have been suppported with VADs for up to 3 months. Since the last "permanent" implantation in 1985, the TAH has been used only in a bridge-to-transplantation capacity. Clinical data from the J-7 TAH bridge-to-transplant patient population show that there is a relatively high percentage of thromboembolic and infectious complications. The incidence of thromboembolism with the TAH ranges from 15% to 35% depending on the categorization of injury. In a recent review of 20 TAH implants, it was noted that 3 patients suffered CVAs.[32] These 3 were all patients with permanent implants who were on various anticoagulation regimens of heparin, warfarin, dipyridamole, and aspirin, or some combination thereof. Four additional patients suffered transient ischemic attacks, which may have been due to microembolization. While thrombus formation within the ventricles themselves is rare, it is not unusual to see circular thrombus in the area of the prosthetic valves and aortic and pulmonary artery quick-connects.[33] Most of the pulsatile assist device systems recommend using a mode of operation that utilizes a complete filling and complete emptying of the blood sac. The output of a VAD is usually regulated by volume rather than rate. In contrast, the TAH is regulated by rate rather than volume, and seldom, except for possibly when the patient is ambulatory, does each ventricle completely fill and empty on each beat. This difference in the washing of the blood sacs could play a role in thrombus formation. Most investigators begin anticoagulation therapy in patients who have the J-7 TAH implanted within 24 hours of insertion. In the operating room, the heparin is reversed with protamine and the patient is watched until his chest tube drainage decreases to an acceptable level. At this point, a continuous infusion of heparin is begun. Dipyridamole may also be used if platelet deaggregation is desired. Once the patient is able to take oral medications, warfarin and dipyridamole may be administered.

Recently, there has been reported a high incidence of infectious complications after cardiac transplantation in patients who have had Symbion artificial hearts implanted. Six of the seven deaths from the University of Pittsburgh occurred as a result of infection.[34] Griffith et al.[34] postulate that removing the natural heart and replacing it with a TAH leaves a space within the mediastinum that cannot be effectively treated with antibiotics and is therefore susceptible to infection. Another disadvantage of removing the natural heart in patients with biventricular failure is that by doing so, the possibility that the patient's heart could recover is eliminated. For this reason, it is considered unwise to treat patients with postcardiotomy cardiogenic shock with placement of a TAH. Rather, biventricular assist devices should be implanted, thus giving the patient's heart the possibility of recovering. Patients with chronic cardiomyopathy and biventricular failure, who have been accepted for cardiac transplantation, are suitable candidates for placement of a TAH.

Management Techniques

Type of Support Required

An important factor in determining which mechanical support device to implant is based on the type of ventricular failure present. In early experimental and clinical trials, the primary concern was mechanical support of the left ventricle. Investigators believed that pharmacologic support would be sufficient to treat associated right ventricular failure.[9, 20] It was soon recognized that primary right ventricular failure can occur in spite of reasonable left ventricular function. In some instances, biventricular failure may not be recognized early in the course of circulatory support.[35] The problem with right ventricular failure in patients undergoing left ventricular bypass was emphasized by Parr et al.,[36] who subsequently described the use of a right VAD as a primary means of support. Since that time, biventricular assist devices have been applied successfully.[35, 37, 38]

It was originally thought that the incidence of biventricular failure would be higher in patients with cardiomyopathy than in patients with ischemic disease. However, there are clear instances of isolated and bilateral ventricular failure in patients with both ischemic and nonischemic cardiomyopathy. The etiology of the heart failure has not been useful in determining the need for biventricular support. To date, hemodynamic criteria are the most useful in determining the type of support required. The atrium with the highest pressure usually indicates the ventricle with predominant failure. However, isolated circulatory support for either the right or left side may "unmask" failure of the other ventricle. It is not unusual to find that after the establishment of left ventricular bypass in a patient who apparently has satisfactory right ventricular function, right-sided heart failure ensues and the patient deteriorates and eventually dies.[35] This phenomenon can be expected to occur approximately 50% to 60% of the time and can be corrected by the use of biventricular mechanical support. It is imperative that the type of support required be determined before deciding which support device is to be used. If there is severe biventricular failure in a patient already selected for cardiac transplantation who deteriorates, a TAH is appropriate. If there is satisfactory right ventricular function and left ventricular dysfunction, a left VAD or LVAS should be used. If the patient develops right ventricular failure after insertion of the left VAD, then biventricular assist devices should be implanted. Since several devices mentioned in the chapter are not designed for right ventricular support, another type of device must be used.

Operation for Insertion

Site.—The more complex systems require insertion in the operating room, usually with CPB and routine cardiac surgical equipment. Patients who deteriorate in the ICU, the emergency room, or the cardiac catheterization laboratory can be placed on simpler circulatory support systems rapidly without the need for a sternotomy (see Table 1). A system for placement of groin cannulas can be employed. Regardless of whether emergency support is established by peripheral cannulation or transseptal techniques, it is doubtful that such systems can be maintained over the period required to obtain a donor heart or until the native heart recovers. Unless a donor heart is immediately available for transplantation, these patients should have a more definitive system inserted.

Incision.—The incision used depends on the selection of the device to be inserted. The peripheral cannulating systems allowing for rapid support require percutaneous techniques or a cutdown, while more complex systems require sternotomy and CPB. In some cases, perfusion may need to be initiated with femorofemoral cannulation, particularly when the patient has undergone a previous sternotomy or is in profound shock. The need for repeated sternotomy for removal of the device and/or cardiac transplantation does not present an inordinately high risk of infection or wound complications. The centrifugal and roller pumps are currently most often used in conjunction with standard CPB cannulas and tubing, which can be placed into the great vessels or cardiac chambers with simple purse-string sutures. The paracorporeal and implantable pumps all require that grafts be sutured to the pump outflow vessel. Problems may arise if the patient has had previous coronary bypass grafts. Occasionally, the device outflow graft must be sutured to the innominate artery or to an unusual site on the ascending aorta.

Several devices can be cannulated to either the left atrium or left ventricle (see Table 1). If it appears that the patient's heart is irreversibly damaged and that transplantation will be required, it is usually preferable to use left ventricular cannulation. The pulsatile pumps seem to fill better from a left ventricle that contracts to fill the pump chamber actively rather than allowing it to fill from the atrium. Whether using atrial or ventricular pump inflow, paracorporeal pneumatic pumps require low levels of vacuum to provide adequate pump filling. Left ventricular cannulas usually require less vacuum than atrial cannulas. Left ventricular cannulation is often difficult in patients after cardiotomy or in those who have acute MI shock and small left ventricles. This has rarely been a problem with cardiac transplant recipients since most of them have dilated left ventricular chambers.

The device should be positioned in such a way that the patient is able to be mobile to facilitate recovery. Paracorporeal pumps allow placement on the abdominal wall. For placement of the Novacor LVAS, we use a single incision extending through the sternum and beyond the umbilicus. We incise the rectus sheath on both sides of the linea alba and dissect the rectus muscle anterior to the posterior rectus sheath, creating a large pocket for the pump. This incision has the advantage of providing muscle layers to cover the pump and avoids problems related to placement inside the peritoneal cavity. Positioning of the Symbion artificial heart has been an important consideration in permanent recipients, as well as candidates for cardiac transplantation. The J-7 (100-cc) TAH can present considerable problems for smaller patients or those with a small anteroposterior thoracic diameter. The development ofthe J-7-70 (70-cc) TAH has facilitated the placement of this device, particularly in smaller men and women. A recent study suggests that the J-7 or J-7-70 device may be used in virtually all adult potential cardiac transplant recipients.[39] It is now our policy to attempt to close the sternum in all patients who have mechanical support devices implanted. This allows for mobilization during the period awaiting transplantation or recovery and limits bleeding from the sternal edges. Extracorporeal membrane oxygenation (ECMO) systems that require a cutdown of the femoral vessels should have the skin closed around the cannulas.

Anticoagulation

The need for anticoagulants with circulatory assist devices complicates the patient's course. Systems using the percutaneous femorofemoral cannulation that employ oxygenators in the circuit obviously require continuous heparinization. Centrifugal and roller pumps placed through sternotomy incisions have been used without anticoagulants by some investigators.[19] However, most investigators who use various centrifugal devices have identified the presence of fibrin in the pump heads in some patients, although thromboembolism has not been a common problem. Currently, we believe that patients treated with centrifugal pumps should be anticoagulated with heparin as soon as the initial bleeding from the operation has subsided. The Pierce-Donachy VAD, however, can be used without heparin for approximately 1 week as long as the flow is maintained above 3 L/min. Patients receiving the Novacor LVAS before transplantation have almost all received some type of anticoagulation, usually a continuous heparin protocol. Since this device employs bovine pericardialvalves, it may be that anticoagulation with heparin is not necessary. However, our current regimen consists of treatment with heparin or warfarin and dipyridamole after 1 week. In four patients maintained at our hospital for more than 50 days (two Novacor, two Thoratec), we were able to change to a regimen of oral warfarin and dipyridamole, during which time there was no evidence to suggest thromboembolic events. The anticoagulation regimen required with the Symbion device is still not completely defined, nor is it entirely established for any of these devices. In the initial experiences with the J-7, DeVries[30] employed a generous heparinization schedule along with aspirin and dipyridamole. This regimen often resulted in bleeding, which led to several complications. Currently, most investigators using the Symbion TAH use continuous heparinization. Aspirin is not usually given because of the danger of bleeding at the time of reoperation. Thromboembolism has been a problem in several patients with this device, but measures are being taken to prevent thromboemboli by more intensive anticoagulation regimens and by design modifications. Unfortunately, with the possible exception of the Novacor LVAS, none of the systems described in this chapter can be relied on to function for more than a few weeks without the threat of thromboembolism, unless some type of anticoagulation regimen is employed.

Regulation of Device

The primary goal of assistance is to establish perfusion as soon as possible to reverse ischemic changes of the vital organs. A minimum value of 2 L/sq m/min of systemic flow is imperative to hope for a successful outcome, but it is desirable to maintain higher flows. The drive parameters vary depending on the device employed. Nonpulsatile centrifugal and roller pumps are driven at rates that produce optimal flow without regard to the patient's intrinsic cardiac rate. However, if the patient's own heart is contributing a significant percentage of the cardiac output, it may be possible to use assist device flows in the range of 2.5 to 3 L/min, particularly with the centrifugal device. Paracorporeal and implantable VADs can be operated in either asynchronous or synchronous modes. In general, the pumps should be adjusted to maintain systemic flow at greater than 2 L/sq m/min. Left and right atrial pressures are maintained in the range of 10 to 15 mm Hg and mean systemic blood pressure is maintained at 65 to 80 mm Hg.

The use of biventricular assist devices was initially feared to present difficult problems of synchronization of the left and right pumps, but this has not been an important clinical problem. It should usually be anticipated that left ventricular flow will exceed right ventricular flow by 500 to 1,000 ml/min because of the return of bronchial flow to the left ventricle. When using paracorporeal pumps, the right and left pumps are usually run in a volume or fill-to-empty mode. Regardless of which drive parameters are employed, synchronization of the pumps to the natural heart is not necessary. The Symbion TAH cannot work in synchrony with a natural heart since the ventricles have been removed.

Clinical Problems

Biventricular Failure

The presence of biventricular failure and the method of treatment are important determinants of survival. Biventricular failure may occur in patients who have sustained an MI of the left and right ventricle or the left ventricle and the intraventricular septum, or in patients with global ischemia. The early recognition and treatment of right ventricular failure is essential to the success of ventricular assistance. Representative of the concern of right ventricular failure is the capability of most of these systems also to provide right ventricular support. Three systems that cannot provide some degree of right-sided heart support are the Elecath left atrial–femoral artery system, the Thermedics LVAS, and the Novacor LVAS.

The development of right ventricular failure in patients with apparently isolated left ventricular failure who received only left ventricular support is still not completely understood. Farrar et al.[40] studied patients undergoing routine coronary bypass operations by measuring right ventricular function shortly after instituting left ventricular bypass. They could identify no evidence that left ventricular bypass induced right ventricular failure. One of the possible explanations for right ventricular failure during left ventricular bypass is the development of progressively increasing pulmonary vascular resistance in patients after cardiotomy.[35] In spite of the fact that many investigators agree that right ventricular failure is an important consideration of mechanical support, few believe that all patients requiring mechanical support should receive biventricular support devices. A prerequisite for initiating left ventricular support should be the ability to provide right ventricular support if needed.

Infection

Clinically, there have been few infections reported that have been a direct result of VADs that have been implanted for less than 1 week.[41] As one would expect, the percentage of infectious complications related to the assist device increases with the duration of the implant.[42] Most infections related to long-term support are associated with percutaneous cannulas or drive lines. It seems likely that external systems that have percutaneous cannulas introduce an added risk of infection, especially in such critically ill patients. Multiple transfusions, the need to be reexplored for bleeding, the presence of numerous pressure-monitoring catheters for periods of up to 2 weeks, and extended time (10 days to 2 weeks) on a ventilator and in bed are major contributors to infectious complications in patients requiring mechanical circulatory support. It has been argued that implantable devices would cause fewer infections than paracorporeal systems because they may eliminate the need for percutaneous cannulas. At this time, however, implantable devices require percutaneous power cables or pneumatic drivelines, which also communicate with the mediastinum.

Bleeding

Bleeding continues to be a major area of concern among investigators using mechanical circulatory support. Although frequently not fatal, bleeding contributes to the development of several other complications, including renal failure and pulmonary congestion. Coagulation disorders are usually similar to the alterations that occur following CPB. These coagulation abnormalities may resolve during the time the device is in place. The patients often have thrombocytopenia during the first week the pump is in place, requiring platelet transfusions as often as once per day. Fibrinogen is usually decreased initially but returns to normal levels after approximately 3 to 4 days. The effects of mechanical circulatory support on antithrombin III and other hemostatic variables is being investigated.[43] On the whole, most patients do not appear to have disseminated intravascular coagulopathy. Instead, they have decreased platelet and fibrinogen levels, resulting in oozing from multiple cannulation sites. Patients with support devices that do not require heparinization usually stop bleeding within 24 hours of insertion of the device. Patients on systems that require continuous heparinization may never completely stop bleeding, and this is often a factor in determining the rate at which the patient is weaned from the device. More recently, however, thrombostatic agents such as fibrin glue, decreased CPB times, and earlier initiation of circulatory support have resulted in a decreased incidence and severity of bleeding complications.

Renal Failure

The etiology of renal failure in patients with mechanical circulatory support devices is often elusive.[44] There is no doubt that the period of hypoperfusion before device insertion, long CPB times, and extensive transfusions contribute to renal insufficiency. However, in many clinical circumstances, renal dysfunction would be expected to be temporary, reversing itself once adequate cardiac output and renal blood flow were reestablished. Unfortunately, this has not proved to be the case in many patients with assist devices. It is not uncommon for patients to develop renal failure that worsens despite the fact that the assist device is in place. Although ultrafiltration and hemodialysis help to maintain fluid balance, blood urea nitrogen (BUN) levels and creatinine levels within a reasonable range, the renal failure often progresses and is sometimes unresponsive to treatment. Many patients who suffer acute renal failure are unable to be weaned from the assist device owing to volume overload. However, if the patient's heart recovers and the kidneys are the only injured organ, long-term hemodialysis may prove to be effective. If treated early enough, it is possible to support patients adequately with only ultrafiltration rather than hemodialysis. During the first week of ultrafiltration, BUN, creatinine, and serum potassium levels do not rise to dangerous levels, and the prime concern during this period is the removal of fluid. However, if renal failure continues past 1 to 2 weeks, it usually becomes necessary to perform hemodialysis. This is often technically difficult in critically ill patients because they respond to hemodialysis with a decrease in blood pressure and cardiac output. For this reason, a continuous hemodialysis system appears to work best with this type of patient. Hemodialysis or ultrafiltration that requires cannulation of the femoral vessels is often detrimental to the patients because it immobilizes them and requires additional anticoagulation.

Weaning

Weaning the patient from a circulatory support device actually begins shortly after the device is inserted and functioning. As soon as possible, one should try to decrease the amount of inotropic drugs the patient is receiving. Weaning of pharmacologic support should continue until the dosage is approximately 2 to 3 μg/kg/min of dopamine and 0.01 μg/kg/min of isoproterenol. Low-dose vasodilators are also frequently necessary. For the first 24 hours of support, the patient is maintained with high flows in an attempt to keep the right and left atrial pressures at approximately 12 to 15 mm Hg and a mean aortic pressure at 70 to 75 mm Hg. Flows with atrial cannulation rarely exceed 5 L/min, and the average flow is approximately 4 L/min. Flows with peripheral cannulation systems are generally lower, usually 3 to 4 L/min.

Approximately 24 hours after implantation, pump on–pump off data should be obtained. With the device temporarily turned off, left and right atrial pressure, pulmonary artery pressures, systemic pressure, cardiac output, and mixed venous oxygen saturation should be measured and compared with similar data obtained with the device on.[45] Once the patient is able to maintain a mean aortic pressure above 70 mm Hg, left and right atrial pressure less than 20 mm Hg, and a cardiac index greater than 2 L sq m/min with the VAD off, the weaning begins. At this point, the ventricle has usually recovered such that there is visible ventricular ejection, as noted on the systemic pressure trace. If the patient is not receiving continuous heparin infusion before beginning the weaning process, a heparin infusion to prolong the activated partial thromboplastin time to 1½ times baseline is started. Depending on the system used, the flow should be gradually decreased.

If the patient is able to maintain the preweaning hemodynamic criteria with a low dose of inotropic drugs, the device is ready to be removed. Moreover, depending on the type of device used, echocardiograms and nuclear MUGA scans can be performed to evaluate ventricular recovery. In our experience, an ejection fraction greater than 30% with the assist device off has been a reliable indicator that myocardial recovery has taken place sufficiently for the patient to survive without the assist device. If after 7 to 10 days the patient cannot maintain the hemodynamics mentioned above with the pump off, transplantation should be considered.

Discussion

The rationale for the use of temporary circulatory support devices is to stabilize the patient, thus allowing time for further treatment (surgery, transplantation, or weaning after recovery). During the critical period following the development of cardiogenic shock, there are two primary considerations: the pumping ability of the heart and the maintenance of satisfactory perfusion to the vital organs. Circulatory support devices affect these areas profoundly and favorably, thus allowing for the survival of patients who would not otherwise survive. While some patients have myocardial injuries severe enough to preclude survival without transplantation, some of them have reversible impairment of ventricular function. Since current diagnostic techniques do not allow precise differentiation of these patients, the overall survival rate is not likely to exceed 70% to 75%. However, over the past several years, technical advances and increased clinical experience have resulted in improved survival rates. It is not apparent that the sooner a firm decision is made to proceed with insertion of a device, the less cardiac and vital organ damage occurs from prolonged periods of cardiogenic shock.

For this reason, systems that allow rapid insertion in areas of the hospital other than the operating room are especially useful. These devices can provide rapid stabilization of patients by avoiding the delay required to reach the operating room. The methods of percutaneous venoarterial ECMO and the transseptal cannulation technique would be well suited to the cardiac catheterization laboratory. However, transseptal cannulation should not be attempted in other areas of the hospital. The patient who suddenly deteriorates in the emergency room or coronary care unit should probably undergo percutaneous femoral placement. If this is not possible, perfusion by femoral cutdown can be accomplished within 10 to 15 minutes. The postcardiotomy patient who deteriorates in the ICU is probably best managed by reopening the sternotomy and placing cannulas into the aorta and right atrium by bypass with the centrifugal or roller pump. Of the systems discussed, the paracorporeal and implantable pumps are the systems that wouuld be least optimal for placement in the ICU, particularly if left ventricular bypass is required. If one of these more sophisticated devices is to be placed, immediate stabilization with one of the simpler systems such as femorofemoral ECMO can be performed and the patient subsequently transferred to the operating room. Also, after placement on one of the rapid insertion systems, the patient could be evaluated during a period of stabilization. For example, a patient placed on femorofemoral ECMO could be stabilized and then taken to the cardiac catheterization laboratory, where a cardiac catheterization could be performed. Additional testing such as an echocardiogram and nuclear MUGA scan could also be performed to evaluate the reversibility of myocardial damage. If the patient appears to have reversible cardiac damage, then she should be taken to the operating room for an operation or placement of a temporary VAD. If the damage is considered irreversible and the patient is determined to be a cardiac transplant candidate, an appropriate method of long-term circulatory support, such as a VAD or TAH, should be considered. Because of the possibility of such a period of patient evaluation, any system that uses a pump oxygenator should incorporate a membrane oxygenator to reduce the degree of trauma to blood components.

Perhaps one of the most significant lessons we have learned is the frequency and importance of biventricular failure. The overall results in patients requiring biventricular support and receiving only univentricular support after cardiac operations has been discouraging.[35] However, with improved understanding over the last several years in the importance of providing biventricular support for patients with biventricular failure, the survival rate is improving. With the exception of the Thermedics LVAS, Novacor LVAS, and the Elecath (transseptal) system, all the pumps mentioned in this article have the capability of providing some degree of biventricular support. The best results may be expected in patients with isolated left ventricular failure, but the number of patients with this more favorable condition has proved to be less than previously expected.

Another important factor leading to improved results has been the use of atrial rather than ventricular cannulation. Clinical experience suggests that left atrial cannulation is simpler and more effective than left ventricular cannulation. Left ventricular apex cannulation damages an already impaired left ventricle and contributes to bleeding complications. Often ventricular cannulas do not drain well in patients with small left ventricles such as those that have suffered an acute MI. Left atrial cannulation avoids most of these problems. Left ventricular cannulation has been used successfully in patients with left ventricles enlarged owing to cardiomyopathy. These bridge-to-transplant patients do not suffer from loss of ventricular mass since their ventricles are removed at the time of transplantation. A classic argument in favor of left ventricular cannulation has been the capability to decompress the left ventricle and rest the heart to promote healing. Several animal laboratory experiments have demonstrated the superiority of left ventricular over left atrial cannulation for decompressing the left ventricle and reducing MI size.[46, 47] However, in actual practice, survival rates of patients with postoperative ventricular failure treated with atrial cannulating devices is superior to rates of those receiving left ventricular cannulating devices.

The paracorporeal and implantable LVASs, along with the three centrifugal pumps mentioned, have the potential to provide complete support of the left ventricle and adequate cardiac output without ventricular ejection. The roller pumps and ECMO systems are usually considered partial unloading systems, while the left atrial and femoral systems clearly provide only partial unloading support. However, complete unloading is not the primary goal, and the more important consideration is to provide sufficient perfusion to vital organs to prevent irreversible injury. At the same time, ventricular unloading may be important in patients with acute MI shock. It is agreed that complete unloading is not accomplished with atrial cannulation, so some investigators believe it is advantageous to pass the left atrial cannulas across the mitral valve into the left ventricle. One indication for such a method of more complete unloading is the presence of left ventricular thrombus, which may be less likely to propagate if the blood is continuously washed out of the left ventricle. Since the primary goal of clinical experiences to date has been therapeutic rather than experimental, it is not surprising that the effects of these assist devices on ventricular function have not been systematically studied, except for estimates of hemodynamic recovery using pump on–pump off measurements.

The effects of systems that use femoral cannulation for unloading the ventricle is unknown. It is questionable whether femoral cannulation systems lower myocardial oxygen consumption and decrease left ventricular pressure to a significant degree. Therefore, in patients who have suffered an acute MI, such systems may be ineffective by only providing adequate perfusion and not allowing for myocardial recovery.[48] This supports the concept that the system should be used as only a temporary stabilization technique until a more efficient and safer method of mechanical circulatory support can be initiated.

Conclusion

Mechanical circulatory support has proved to be an effective treatment for patients with severe ventricular failure. Although assist devices have been available for nearly 30 years, recent improvements in survival rates have sparked widespread interest. Centers that treat a large number of patients with cardiogenic shock realize that some of these patients will not respond to treatment with IABPs and conventional therapy. For this reason, many institutions that perform open heart operations are obtaining commercially available and investigational devices to provide these patients with a more efficient form of circulatory support.

Systems that utilize peripheral cannulation and provide rapid stabilization of the patient are becoming more widely used. These are short-term devices that ideally should be used only to stabilize the patient and allow for a short period of evaluation (24 hours). In addition to these systems that provide a method of rapid resuscitation, a system that would provide safer and more efficient support for longer durations (7 to 14 days) is also needed. Patients in acute MI shock could be supported with devices until myocardial recovery occurs or until they are stabilized and are determined to be operative candidates. They would then undergo surgical intervention at the appropriate time. More clinical experience is needed with the acute MI shock group to determine to what degree the myocardial damage is reversible and to better define patient selection criteria. The value of mechanical support devices has been established in the bridge-to-transplant and postcardiotomy groups; survival statistics are better than most investigators had anticipated and should improve with experience and better devices.

References

1. Dennis C, Spreng DS, Nelson GE, et al: Development of a pump-oxygenator to replace the heart and lungs: An apparatus applicable to human patients, and application to one case. *Ann Surg* 1951; 134:709.
2. Gibbon JH Jr: Application of a mechanical heart and lung apparatus to cardiac surgery. *Minn Med* 1954; 37:171.
3. Stuckey JH, Newman MM, Dennis C, et al: The use of the heart lung machine in selected cases of acute myocardial infarction. *Surg Forum* 1957; 8:342.
4. Spencer FC, Eiseman B, Trinkle JK, et al: Assisted circulation for cardiac failure following intracardiac surgery with cardiopulmonary bypass. *J Thorac Cardiovasc Surg* 1965; 49:56.
5. Debakey ME: Left ventricular bypass pump for cardiac assistance: Clinical experience. *Am J Cardiol* 1971; 27:3.
6. Kantrowitz A, Tjonneland S, Freed PS, et al: Initial clinical experience with intra-aortic balloon pumping in cardiogenic shock. *JAMA* 1968; 203:135.
7. McEnany MT, Kay HR, Buckley MJ, et al: Clinical experience with intra-aortic balloon pump support in 728 patients. *Circulation* 1977; 58:124.
8. Norman JC, Cooley DA, Igo SR, et al: Prognostic indices for survival during postcardiotomy intra-aortic balloon pumping. *J Thorac Cardiovasc Surg* 1977; 74:709.
9. Holub DA, Hibbs CW, Sturm JT, et al: Clinical trials of the abdominal left ventricular assist device (ALVAD): Progress report. *Cardiovas Dis* 1979; 6:359.
10. Bernhard WF, Poirier V, LaFarge CG, et al: A new method for temporary left ventricular bypass: Preclinical appraisal. *J Thorac Cardiovasc Surg* 1975; 70:880.
11. Pierce WS, Brighton JA, O'Bannon W, et al: Complete left ventricular bypass with a paracorporeal pump: Design and evaluation. *Ann Surg* 1974; 180:418.
12. Pennington DG, Bernhard WF, Golding LR, et al: Long-term follow-up of postcardiotomy patients with profound cardiogenic shock treated with ventricular assist devices. *Circulation* 1984; 72:216.
13. Pennington DG, Merjavy JP, Swartz MT, et al: Clinical experience with a centrifugal pump ventricular assist device. *Trans Am Soc Artif Intern Organs* 1982; 28:93.
14. Golding LR, Jacobs G, Groves LK, et al: Clinical results of mechanical support of the failing left ventricle. *J Thorac Cardiovasc Surg* 1982; 83:597.
15. Rose DM, Laschinger J, Grossi E, et al: Experimental and clinical results with a simplified left heart assist device for treatment of profound ventricular dysfunction. *World J Surg* 1985; 9:11.
16. Rose DM, Colvin SB, Culliford AT, et al: Long-term survival with partial left heart bypass following perioperative myocardial infarction and shock. *J Thorac Cardiovasc Surg* 1982; 83:483.
17. Pennock JL, Pierce WS, Wisman CB, et al: Survival and complications following ventricular assist pumping for cardiogenic shock. *Ann Surg* 1983; 198:469.
18. Pennington DG, Samuels LD, Williams G, et al: Experience with the Pierce-Donachy ventricular assist device in postcardiotomy patients with cardiogenic shock. *World J Surg* 1985; 9:37.
19. Magovern GJ, Park SB, Maher TD: Use of a centrifugal pump without anticoagulants for postoperative left ventricular assist. *World J Surg* 1985; 9:25.
20. Bernhard WF, Berger RL, Stetz JP, et al: Temporary left ventricular bypass: Factors affecting patient survival. *Circulation* 1978; 60:131.

21. Ischinger T (ed): Practice of Coronary Angioplasty. New York, Springer-Verlag New York, p 246.
22. Pennington DG, McBride LR, Swartz MT, et al: The effect of perioperative myocardial infarction on survival of postcardiotomy patients supported with ventricular assist devices. Circulation, in press.
23. Pennington DG: Circulatory support pre-transplant, in Wallwork J (ed): Cardiac and Cardiopulmonary Transplantation. New York, Grune & Stratton, in press.
24. Farrar DJ, Hill JD, Gray LA, et al: Heterotopic prosthetic ventricles as a bridge to cardiac transplantation: A multicenter study in 29 patients. N Engl J Med 1988; 318:333.
25. Kanter KR, Swartz MT, Pennington DG, et al: Emergency extracorporeal membrance oxygenation (ECMO) for cardiopulmonary resuscitation, abstracted. Heart Transplant 1988; 7:75.
26. Laschinger JC, Cunningham JN, Catinella FP, et al: "Pulsatile" left atrial–femoral artery bypass: A new method of preventing extension of myocardial infarction. Arch Surg 1983; 118:965.
27. Phillips SJ: Percutaneous cardiopulmonary bypass and innovations in clinical counterpulsation. Crit Care Clin 1986; 2:297–318.
28. Pennington DG, Merjavy JP, Codd JE, et al: Extracorporeal membrane oxygenation for patients with cardiogenic shock. Circulation 1983; 70:130.
29. Frazier OH, Painvin GA, Urrutia CO, et al: Mechanical circulatory support: Clinical experience at the Texas Heart Institute. Heart Transplant 1983; 2:299.
30. DeVries WC: The permanent artificial heart: Four case reports. JAMA 1988; 259:849.
31. Kunin CM, Dobbins JJ, Melo JC, et al: Infectious complications in four long-term recipients of the Jarvik-7 artificial heart. JAMA 1988; 259:860.
32. Joyce LD, Johnson KE, Pierce WS, et al: Summary of the world experience with clinical use of total artificial heart as heart support devices. Heart Transplant 1986; 5:229.
33. Levinson MM, Smith RG, Cork R, et al: Three recent cases of the total artificial heart before transplantation. Heart Transplant 1986; 5:215.
34. Griffith BP, Kormos RL, Hardesty RL, et al: The artificial heart: Infection-related morbidity and its effect on transplantation. Ann Thorac Surg 1988; 45:409.
35. Pennington DG, Merjavy JP, Swartz MT, et al: The importance of biventricular failure in patients with postoperative cardiogenic shock. Ann Thorac Surg 1985; 39:16.
36. Parr GVS, Pierce WS, Rosenberg G, et al: Right ventricular failure after repair of left ventricular aneurysm. J Thorac Cardiovasc Surg 1980; 80:79.
37. Turina MT, Bosio R, Senning A: Paracorporeal artificial heart in postoperative heart failure. Artif Organs 1978; 2:273.
38. Park SB, Liebler GA, Burkholder JA, et al: Mechanical support of the failing heart. Ann Thorac Surg 1986; 42:627.
39. Jarvik RK, DeVries WC, Semb KHB, et al: Surgical positioning of the Jarvik-7 total artificial heart. Heart Transplant 1980; 5:184.
40. Farrar DJ, Compton PG, Hershon JJ, et al: Right ventricular function in an operating room model of mechanical left ventricular assistance and its effects in patients with depressed left ventricular function. Circulation 1985; 72:1279.
41. McBride LR, Ruzevich SA, Pennington DG, et al: Infectious complications associated with ventricular assist device support. Trans Am Soc Artif Intern Organs 1987; 33:201.

42. McBride LR, Galbraith TA, Pennington DG, et al: Long-term bridging to cardiac transplantation, abstracted. *Heart Transplant* 1988; 7:76.
43. Joist JH, Pennington DG: Platelet reactions with artificial surfaces. *Trans Am Soc Artif Intern Organs* 1987; 33:341.
44. Kanter KR, Swartz MT, Pennington DG, et al: Renal failure in patients with ventricular assist devices. *Trans Am Soc Artif Intern Organs* 1987; 33:426.
45. Termuhlen DF, Swartz MT, Pennington DG, et al: Predictors for weaning patients from ventricular assist devices (VADs). *Trans Am Soc Artif Intern Organs* 1987; 33:683.
46. Pennock JL, Pae WE, Pierce WS, et al: Reduction of myocardial infarct size: Comparison between left atrial and left ventricular bypass. *Circulation* 1979; 59:275.
47. Laks H, Hahn JW, Blair O, et al: Cardiac assistance and infarct size: Left atrial-to-aortic vs left ventricular-to-aortic bypass. *Surg Forum* 1976; 27:226.
48. Bavaria JE, Ratcliffe MB, Gupta KB, et al: Changes in left ventricular systolic wall stress during biventricular circulatory assistance. *Ann Thorac Surg* 1988; 45:526.

Cardiovascular Grafts and Synthetic Materials

Lester R. Sauvage, M.D.

Department of Surgery, University of Washington School of Medicine, Hope
Heart Institute, Providence Medical Center, Seattle, Washington

Today there are many manufacturers presenting a wide variety of effective cardiovascular prostheses for the surgical patient. This was certainly not true when I was in medical school (1944–1948) or for many years afterward. I still remember the thrill I experienced in those early years reading about the great accomplishments of Drs. Gross, Hufnagel, Potts, Bailey, Harker, DeBakey, Cooley, and Szilagyi. These men were the giants who forged a path in the wilderness for the rest of us to follow. Of these I am most indebted to Dr. Robert E. Gross, with whom I had the opportunity to spend 2 years at the Boston Children's Hospital during 1956 to 1958.

In this chapter I will not try to analyze all types of prostheses but instead will present an account of my personal experience in this field. I have been involved in experimental cardiovascular research in a continuous manner since 1950, the first 4 years full-time and the last 33 years on a part-time basis in conjunction with surgical training (4 years) and medical practice (29 years). My thinking, therefore, has evolved from both research and clinical experiences.

At the inception of my clinical practice I had the opportunity simultaneously to begin the development of a surgical research laboratory at the Providence Medical Center in Seattle. In 1958, it was unknown in Seattle for someone in private practice also to have an animal research laboratory at a private hospital. I still remember with deep gratitude the administrator of the Providence Medical Center in those days, Sister Genevieve, S.P., a 75-year-old nun of great vision, who gave me space to begin work in an old home built in 1900 that was owned by the hospital. A $6,000 grant from the Washington State Heart Association provided initial financing in 1959, and it was followed a year later by a $252,000 grant from the John A. Hartford Foundation of New York. The support of Dr. Gross was essential to our receiving the Hartford funds. Additional major grants were subsequently received from the Hartford Foundation. Later, we received substantial support from the National Institutes of Health.

Our initial work in 1958 dealt with the use of pericardium in an intracardiac position and led to the development of an operation called "leaflet advancement for the correction of mitral insufficiency."[1] At the same time we began to study arterial prostheses, an extension of the work I had had the opportunity to initiate during 1952 to 1954 while assigned to the Army Medical Service Graduate School at the Walter Reed Army Medical Center.

I categorize cardiovascular prostheses as either active or passive, depending on whether or not they contribute energy to assist the movement of blood. In this context, intra-aortic balloons, artificial hearts, and heart transplants are classified as active prostheses because they provide energy to assist the movement of blood. On the other hand, prostheses that serve as conduits, patches, partitions, or valves do not contribute energy to move blood and are classified as passive. I further classify passive prostheses into those *in* blood and those *around* blood. In the rest of this discussion I shall focus on my experiences with these passive prostheses.

Passive Prostheses in Blood

Valvular

My personal use of valvular prostheses (Fig 1) goes back to 1963, when I implanted a Starr-Edwards aortic ball valve for the relief of severe aortic stenosis. At that time, Dr. Starr's prostheses were only a few years old, and the basic construction consisted of a metal housing with a porous fabric sewing ring and a silicone elastomer (Silastic) ball.[2] I was impressed, as was the world, with Dr. Starr's and Mr. Lowell Edwards' tremendous contributions to the surgical field. These prostheses were effective and durable.[3] They did have the disadvantage of a long cage that protruded far into the ventricle or up into the aorta, and in some patients with small ventricles the end of the cage could impinge against the septum. Furthermore, in patients with small aortic roots, the ball in the open position could be a major obstacle to blood flow.[4]

Based on extensive studies carried out in calves, we developed an aortic valve (the "V-S-W") and implanted it successfully in several patients with good long-term success.[5-7] This valve embodied what we termed a "guided flow principle."[8] The sewing ring was very small, based on observations of the limitations of healing that we had observed experimentally. We continued valve replacement studies, primarily aortic, during the 1960s, using approximately 500 calves for these studies. We came to the conclusion that in the aortic site pannus ingrowth was capable of extending only 8 to 10 mm from the wall onto a fabric surface.[9] At the same time, the Starr-Edwards totally cloth-covered valve concept was being introduced with the thought that it would solve the problem of thromboembolism by enabling tissue coverage of the total valve. Because of our experimental studies,[10] I was certain this would not work, and unfortunately I was right.[11] The cloth-covered concept for the Starr-Edwards valve was subsequently abandoned. Ball valves continue to be manufactured today, but with a small sewing ring and a bare metal housing. Because of the length of the cage, ball valves have fallen into relative disuse.

The next valve with which I had experience was the old-style Björk-

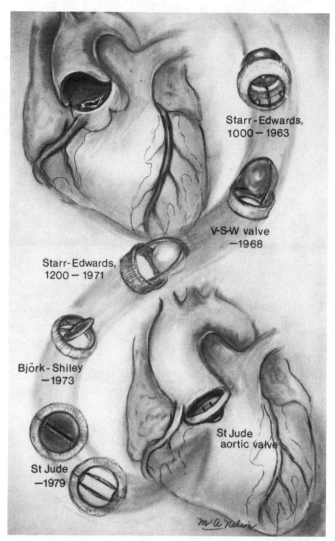

FIG 1.
Chronologic sequence of personal use of prosthetic aortic valves from 1963 to the present.

Shiley,[12-15] first implanting an aortic prosthesis on Nov. 3, 1973. I was very impressed with this valve and generally had good results with it, but felt that the minor orifice was a liability because if thrombus ever started to extend out over it, the disc motion would be severely limited, leading to valve thrombosis; I had this happen in a few instances. For this reason, on July 2, 1979, I switched to the St. Jude valve[16-24] as my mechanical valve of choice and have continued to use it with satisfaction since that time.

I like the St. Jude valve concept because it is a bileaflet valve that opens to provide a very efficient orifice; in addition, the location of the pivoting mechanism is separated from the sewing ring by several millimeters. Concerning durability, since 1979 I have implanted 343 St. Jude valves and have had no instance of mechanical failure.

In 1971, I implanted my first bioprosthetic valve, a Hancock aortic bioprosthesis, experimentally in the calf. In the early days I was very skeptical about this heterograft valve. The first valves were treated with formalin and did not stand up.[25] Warren Hancock then developed the glutaraldehyde-treated porcine valve. I well remember the discussion of these valves at those early meetings as it became obvious that a valve suitable for human use had been developed.[26-29] However, over time calcification and leaflet fracture did occur, but not for 5 or more years in the great majority of instances. Mr. Hancock believed that a fixed ring was better than a malleable ring, and in the early days of bioprosthetic valves his prostheses were favored by a majority of surgeons. I implanted my first Hancock clinical bioprosthetic valve on April 20, 1975, an aortic replacement (Fig 2). I have long believed that the developmental work of Warren Hancock represents one of the great accomplishments of cardiac surgery.

After Hancock had shown that bioprosthetic valves were practical, the Edwards Company, with Alain Carpentier of France, developed the Car-

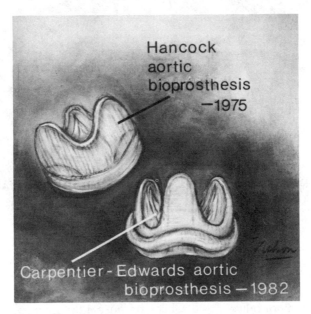

FIG 2.
The historic Hancock bioprosthesis with rigid stent was widely used in the 1970s; however, the Carpentier-Edwards bioprosthesis with flexible stent is now used more frequently.

pentier-Edwards flexible ring bioprosthetic valve.[30-36] Interestingly, after Johnson & Johnson acquired the Hancock Laboratories, the Carpentier-Edwards line of porcine valves progressively took over the dominant market share of the bioprosthetic field. I, too, switched to the Carpentier-Edwards valve and use it primarily for elderly patients requiring aortic valve replacement, in whom anticoagulation would be hazardous (see Fig 2).

The experimental studies that we performed in the calf emphasized the limitations of pannus ingrowth to heal the sewing ring.[10, 11, 37] We further observed experimentally that the best results occurred when we did not implant a large valve that pressed into the tissue but instead implanted one whose base would be washed thoroughly by the ejection of blood both beneath it and through it.[38-40] We have observed that thrombotic complications are rare when these simple relationships between the cardiovascular wall and the valve body are achieved.

Concerning anticoagulation,[41] I have never been an advocate of high-dose warfarin sodium (Coumadin). My preference for 20 years has been low-dose Coumadin to increase the prothrombin time only 3 to 4 seconds. My clinical results have justified this conservative program, and I have seen no reason to change. I believe that most people with the St. Jude valve have come to adopt an approximate 1.5–1 protime elevation over control recommendation. Contrary to the opinion of many, I believe that the bioprosthetic valve in the mitral area is at as great a risk for thromboembolic complications as the St. Jude valve and accordingly anticoagulate my patients who receive these valves. I use a bioprosthetic valve for mitral replacement only when I need its large sewing ring to cover a large denuded area or large areas of calcification that I cannot remove.

Concerning myocardial support, I use moderate hypothermia to 28°C in most instances and either perfuse the isolated root in the case of mitral replacement or use direct coronary cannulation for an aortic replacement. My current technique for myocardial protection is a bit different than most: I begin with high potassium (K20 dropping to K10 as asystole is achieved) at 16°C and follow it with a K10 crystalloid washout at 4°C. I do this because blood supplies oxygen and nutrients best, but in my opinion leaving stagnant blood in the coronaries is injurious because it becomes a "hemic mustard plaster" on the endothelial surface. That is why I wash the cardioplegic (16°C) blood out of the coronaries with a crystalloid washout delivered at 4°C. I repeat this cycle every 20 to 30 minutes.

If the exposure is good and the valve anulus is suitable, I implant mitral prostheses with a running 2-0 Tycron suture. I have done this for years and to my knowledge I have never had a perivalvular leak with a valve so implanted. If the exposure is difficult, I use interrupted sutures, and for aortic valve replacement I always use interrupted sutures of 2-0 Tycron.

Since the introduction of the St. Jude valve, several other valves designed in a similar manner have been introduced that I am sure are very acceptable prostheses. My own bias, however, is to continue to use the St. Jude valve.

Septal Partitions

In my early days of practice in Seattle and continuing through 1979, I was actively involved in pediatric cardiac surgery at the Children's Hospital. However, owing to the growth of my adult cardiovascular surgery practice and the time commitments of directing the research programs of the Hope Heart Institute, I had to withdraw from my work in pediatric surgery.

For closure of septal defects where a patch valve is required, I prefer a graft of autogenous pericardium, even though I have been instrumental in developing a Dacron patch graft for use in the cardiac septa and arterial wall.[42-44] My reason for preferring pericardium for the cardiac septa is that there is two-way healing with the use of such a graft: the graft heals to the implant site and the implant site heals to the graft instead of all the healing coming from the implant site onto the graft. Nonetheless, the patch graft material I developed is often used by my partners in pediatric cardiac surgery for septal closure with excellent results.

The graft that we designed has a velour surface on both sides, lower on one side than the other, but still low even on the higher side. This low (smoothest) side is directed to the left when used as a septal partition. The velour surface of this graft serves to bind fibrin securely to both surfaces, preventing embolization.

Cardiac septal partitions also heal by pannus ingrowth, which is limited to not more than 15 mm. This means that the midportion of a septal patch larger than 3 cm will not heal. However, the central portion of such a patch rarely becomes a source of emboli; instead, it remains surfaced by securely anchored passivated fibrin, which serves as a very effective interface with the blood.

Prostheses Around Arterial Blood

I believe it is an important distinction to consider valves as prostheses in blood with a peripheral attachment, and arterial conduits as grafts around blood (Fig 3). A valve projects into the blood and has only a limited peripheral attachment to the cardiovascular wall at its attachment site, and in like manner an arterial prosthesis has a contact with the host arterial wall only at its anastomotic site. However, the outer wall of the arterial prosthesis is everywhere in contact with the perigraft tissues, while its inner wall is everywhere in contact with blood, in contrast to the valve prosthesis, which is bathed in blood.

Most arterial prostheses have two generic components, a fiber framework for strength and, if the interstices in the fiber framework are rectangular or triangular and are sufficiently large (probably over 200 sq μm), a matrix that fills in the interstices of the framework to render the wall impervious to blood under arterial pressure. If the interstices are very small (probably below 50 to 100 sq μm), the viscosity and surface tension of blood prevent bleeding through these tiny openings.

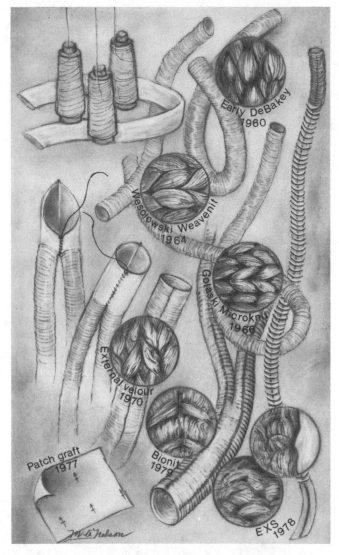

FIG 3.
Chronologic sequence of personal use of knitted Dacron prostheses from 1960 to the present.

Arterial prostheses that require a matrix to prevent loss of blood through their interstices may be classified as macroporous, and if they do not, as microporous. The interstices of microporous grafts are filled with air, while the interstices of macroporous grafts must be filled with an occluding substance either by the surgeon in preclotting (fibrin) or by the manufacturer in processing (albumin or collagen combined with an aldehyde). Polytetrafluoroethylene (PTFE) and tightly woven Dacron prostheses are microporous and do not require a matrix, whereas knitted prostheses do.

A few definitions may be helpful at this point. The abbreviation PTFE, for Teflon, should have an *e* in front of it to signify that in manufacture the Teflon material has been expanded into a microporous open configuration with nodes and connecting filaments (Fig 4,A and B). As time has passed, this *e* designation has been dropped.

Fabric grafts may be of woven or knitted construction (see Fig 4,C to H). The surface of a fabric graft may be relatively smooth or it may be made fuzzy by bringing a yarn bundle composed of texturized filaments to the surface and reducing the tension on this bundle, which allows the filaments to spread, curl, and coil (Fig 5), producing a fuzzy surface referred to as veloured, either externally, internally, or both.

A woven prosthesis is composed of many longitudinal yarn bundles that are interlocked by a single circular bundle that passes over one longitudinal bundle, under the next, over the next, etc. The greater the number of longitudinal yarn bundles per unit distance is and the tighter the circular bundle that binds them together is, the more microporous is the prosthesis. However, if the circular bundle is programmed in manufacture to pass un-

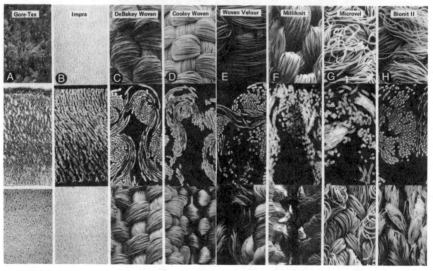

FIG 4.
Photomicrographs of polytetrafluoroethylene and Dacron prostheses. *Top row,* scanning electron microscopy (SEM) of outer surfaces. *Middle row,* light microscopy of longitudinal sections, with flow surface at bottom. *Bottom row,* SEM of inner surfaces. Approximate original magnifications, ×50. (From Sauvage LR: Opportunities and responsibilities in the use of arterial grafts. *Surg Annu* 1984; 16:97, 98, 102; and from Sauvage LR, Davis CC, Smith JC, et al: Development and clinical use of porous Dacron arterial prostheses, in Sawyer PN [ed]: *Modern Vascular Grafts.* New York, McGraw-Hill Book Co, 1987, p 244. Used by permission.)

A

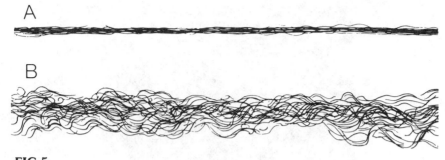

B

FIG 5.
A, texturized Dacron yarn under tension. **B,** texturized Dacron yarn with tension released.

der or over two longitudinal bundles instead of one in a recurring fashion, the tension on these longitudinal bundles is partially released, allowing their texturized filaments to assume a velour configuration, giving rise to the term *woven double velour* (see Fig 4,E). The porosity of the woven double velour graft is increased by the loosening of the structure, making preclotting necessary. However, the preclotting process is expedited by the still low water permeability of the wall (c 500 ml/cm^2/min at 120 mm Hg) and by the velour configuration in the areas of increased permeability. The healing and handling characteristics of this prosthesis are superior to that of tightly woven prostheses. However, negative features of the woven pros-thesis, in addition to the need for preclotting, are reduced strength and a greater tendency of its free edge to fray.

Knitted prostheses are of much looser construction than woven (Fig 4,F to H) and, as a consequence, have better handling characteristics, are eas-ier to suture, and heal better, but must be preclotted to render their walls impervious to the passage of blood. The preclotted knitted or woven dou-ble velour graft should be regarded as a compound prosthesis, partly an autograft of vascular protein (fibrin) forming both surfaces and filling the interstices, and partly synthetic (Dacron) forming a fiber framework lying within the matrix.

Knitted grafts may be constructed by a relatively simple process referred to as weft knitting (Fig 6,A) or by a more complex process referred to as warp knitting (Fig 6,B). The essence of weft knitting is that a seamless tu-bular conduit is formed by one continuous yarn bundle with interlocking loops. The essence of warp knitting is that a double-seamed tubular con-duit is formed by many longitudinal yarn bundles that are interlaced to-gether by interlocking transverse yarn bundles.

The advantages of the weft-knit graft are its uniformity and the absence of seams. The disadvantage of the warp-knit graft is that it is formed from two panels that are joined together by two seams. However, the warp-knit grafts have two salient advantages over the weft-knit: they are stronger and less porous. Because of these features, the warp-knit process is used for the construction of most knitted grafts in use today.

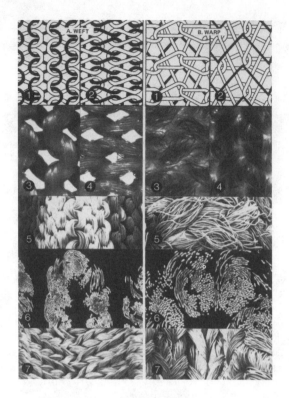

FIG 6.
Photomicrographs and transilluminations illustrating the differences between **(A)** weft-knit (Golaski Microknit), and **(B)** warp-knit (USCI Sauvage Bionit II) Dacron prostheses. *A1, B1,* diagrammatic representation of outer surfaces. *A2, B2,* diagrammatic representation of inner surfaces. *A3, B3,* transillumination of outer surfaces. *A4, B4,* transillumination of inner surfaces. *A5, B5,* scanning electron microscopy (SEM) of outer surfaces. *A6, B6,* light microscopy of longitudinal sections with flow surface at bottom. *A7, B7,* SEM of inner surfaces. Approximate original magnifications, ×50. (From Sauvage LR, Davis CC, Smith JC, et al: Development and clinical use of porous Dacron arterial prostheses, in Sawyer PN [ed]: *Modern Vascular Grafts.* New York, McGraw-Hill Book Co, 1987, pp 229, 244; and from Mathisen SR, Wu H-D, Sauvage LR, et al: The influence of denier and porosity on performance of a warp-knit Dacron arterial prosthesis. *Ann Surg* 1986; 203:383, 384. Used by permission.)

My first clinical experience with arterial prostheses was with the old-style DeBakey knitted prosthesis.[45] The first DeBakey graft that I implanted was in the aortofemoral position, on Nov. 13, 1961. I continued to use this graft in the early years of my practice and found it satisfactory. In the mid-1960s, I began to use the lighter Wesolowski Weavenit prosthesis,[46] which had a 40-needle-per-inch weft-knit construction. However, this graft had such a high porosity that the manufacturer subsequently tried to decrease it by additional heat shrinkage. At that time it was not recognized that this overheating of the graft during manufacture was changing the crystalline structure of the Dacron into a configuration that did not have adequate durability for long-term dimensional stability.[47] Over the next few years, several of these grafts that I had implanted developed localized areas of fiber breakdown with subsequent false aneurysm formation.[47]

The Wesolowski graft, which I liked, was knitted at a higher density than any previous graft, and I reasoned that if we could obtain even higher-density knitting with still lighter yarn the tissue would be able to heal this prosthesis even faster. This led to our development in the middle and later part of the 1960s of a graft we called Microknit.[48] We carried out extensive studies in the descending thoracic aorta of dogs and were horrified to observe that a large number of the animals died between 7 and 35 days of delayed hemorrhage into the pleural space. However, this delayed hemorrhage did not occur in man, indicating that the dog had a higher fibrinolytic capacity. We implanted over 100 of these grafts in patients and in general they worked well, but there was no significant benefit over the old-style DeBakey graft other than that they were easier to suture.[49] They were, however, harder to preclot. On the basis of this experience, I came to the conclusion that there was no further benefit to making even lighter grafts and that the difficulties in preclotting and the consequent dangers of hemorrhage made it unwise to pursue this design further. The conclusion was difficult for me to accept because we had been so enthusiastic about the prospects of this extremely light, high-density graft development.[50]

Out of adversity another development was born, and that was our interest in placing a velour surface on the outside of knitted arterial prostheses for two reasons: first, to provide a filamentous surface for the tissue to adhere to that would serve as a trellis for the ingrowth of cells, and second, to serve as a more efficient mold for preclotting.[51, 52] At the time of our interest in the external velour surface in the middle 1960s, the DeBakey internal velour surface was quite popular. It was my belief that a velour surface belonged on the outside and that the inside of a fabric graft should be kept as smooth as possible. My attitudes in this regard have not changed over the last 20 years. We have shown that an internal velour surface increases fibrin deposition and therefore predisposes to thrombotic complications in small-caliber vessels.[53] There is no doubt that a double velour surface makes preclotting easier than an external velour surface alone. However, proper preclotting of an optimally constructed knitted graft with an external velour surface is quite easily accomplished.[54]

In 1970, an external velour weft-knitted Dacron graft of our design was released by United States Catheter and Instrument Company (USCI; Billerica, Mass), and we implanted it until 1978.[55] Although this graft had many good points, the weft-knit technique would not permit it to be manufactured as a seamless bifurcation graft. I made my own bifurcations by hand during that time and had no technical problems with any of them. These grafts had a water permeability of about 3,000 ml/cm^2/min under a pressure head of 120 mm Hg, and preclotting on occasion could be difficult. In addition, fiber breakdown occurred in a few cases.[47] For these reasons, we decided to develop a graft that was stronger and had a lower porosity. In 1978, we shifted to a warp knit prosthesis called Bionit, manufactured by C. R. Bard (Billerica, Mass), which had a water permeability of about 1,500 ml/cm^2/min and a much stronger wall.

In an effort to decrease the water permeability further, and thus to enhance the ease of preclotting without significant loss of desirable surgical handling characteristics, we carried out extensive studies in the laboratory from 1983 to 1985, leading to the production of the Bionit II prosthesis.[56] This prosthesis has a water permeability of about 1,000 ml/cm^2/min at 120 mm Hg pressure, preclots easily, has desirable physical handling attributes, and has excellent full-wall healing characteristics in the dog and outer wall healing characteristics in humans. I prefer this prosthesis for abdominal aortic bifurcation replacement, for aortofemoral bypass, and for femorofemoral bypass.

I have had comparatively little experience in the thoracic aorta but have found the properly preclotted Bionit II graft satisfactory in the ascending aorta with bypass and in the descending thoracic aorta without bypass. However, until I have obtained greater experience in these areas with the Bionit II, I must continue to recommend use of a tightly woven Dacron graft that has been made more impervious by soaking in an albumin solution and autoclaved at 250°C for 3 minutes.[57−59]

In 1978, with Bard we introduced another innovation in arterial prosthesis development, an externally supported (EXS), noncrimped graft with an external velour surface for use in axillofemoral and lower-extremity bypass (Fig 7).[60−63] In the past year we have shifted from weft-knit to warp-knit construction for these EXS prostheses to achieve lower porosity with greater ease of preclotting and greater strength.

We have found that the EXS prostheses for axillofemoral use have been very successful (Fig 8,A). Patencies for above-knee femoropopliteal bypass have been less satisfactory, but this graft is nonetheless an attractive alternative to the saphenous vein in many instances in this location (see Fig 8,B). However, the EXS and all other synthetic prostheses are clearly inferior to a good saphenous vein for below-knee bypass.

Preclotting is a subject that has long interested me. In 1978, we described a controlled method that has stood the test of time.[54] In brief, this involves wetting the graft with nonheparinized blood and allowing thrombin to form throughout the graft, and then adding nonheparinized blood, which must be handled very rapidly because of the swifness of the reaction of fibrinogen conversion to fibrin and of polymerization to insoluble fibrin. I consider it absolutely essential then to use heparinized blood to inactivate the thrombin by complexing it with the heparin-activated antithrombin III in the heparinized blood and to use a sufficient amount of blood so that all the thrombin is complexed, leaving an excess of heparin-activated antithrombin III on the surface and throughout the wall of the graft to make it truly hypothrombogenic (Fig 9). The porous fabric graft is an incomplete prosthesis when received from the manufacturer because it is only a mold to be used by the surgeon in preclotting to form what I refer to as a "bio-

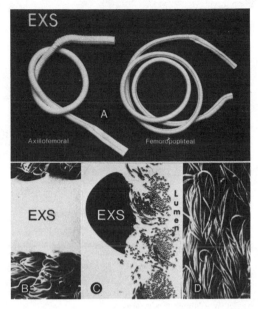

FIG 7.
A, externally supported (EXS) Dacron prostheses for axillofemoral *(left)* and femoropopliteal *(right)* bypass. **B,** scanning electron microscopy (SEM) of outer surface of supported section. **C,** light microscopy of longitudinal section. **D,** SEM of inner surface. Approximate original magnifications, ×50. (From Sauvage LR, Davis CC, Smith JC, et al: Development and clinical use of porous Dacron arterial prostheses, in Sawyer PN [ed]: *Modern Vascular Grafts.* New York, McGraw-Hill Book Co, 1987, p 242. Used by permission.)

synthetic composite of fibrin and Dacron" (Fig 10). I believe this properly preclotted fabric graft is the most sophisticated prosthesis that can be used in a patient today. The blood interfaces with autogenous vascular protein on the inside, as do the perivascular tissues on the outside. This graft is formed of nature's vascular protein, which is the primary sealant for injured vascular surfaces. Admittedly, humans have a limited capacity to endothelialize these prostheses, except by pannus ingrowth closely adjacent to the suture lines. However, if proper hemostasis is present around the graft, perigraft ingrowth to about the midwall depth will occur within 2 months (Fig 11,A). Progression beyond that point is slow and uncertain (Fig 11,B), but the passivated fibrin flow surface of a properly preclotted graft can serve indefinitely if the flow rate across its surface is reasonably rapid. Although I cannot prove it, I believe that if the flow rate that crosses the surface is as much as 6 to 8 ml/cm^2 cross-sectional area per second, then the graft will stay open in patients unless they have a high thrombotic potential.

One of the very important observations in our laboratory has been the work spearheaded by Dr. Svetlana Kaplan, in which she demonstrated the

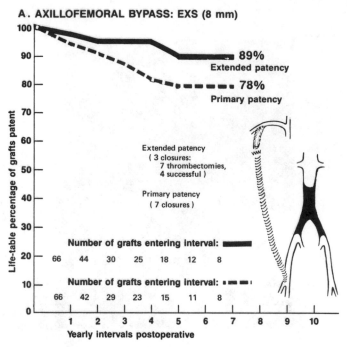

A. AXILLOFEMORAL BYPASS: EXS (8 mm)

89%
Extended patency

78%
Primary patency

Extended patency
(3 closures:
7 thrombectomies,
4 successful)

Primary patency
(7 closures)

Number of grafts entering interval: ▬▬▬
66   44   30   25   18   12   8

Number of grafts entering interval: ▪▬ ▬▬ ▬▪
66   42   29   23   15   11   8

Yearly intervals postoperative

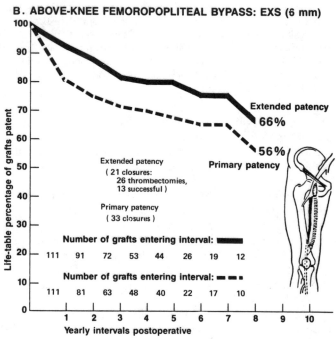

B. ABOVE-KNEE FEMOROPOPLITEAL BYPASS: EXS (6 mm)

Extended patency
66%

56%
Primary patency

Extended patency
(21 closures:
26 thrombectomies,
13 successful)

Primary patency
(33 closures)

Number of grafts entering interval: ▬▬▬
111   91   72   53   44   26   19   12

Number of grafts entering interval: ▬▬ ▬▪
111   81   63   48   40   22   17   10

Yearly intervals postoperative

FIG 8.
Life tables illustrating clinical performance of the externally supported (EXS) graft in the **(A)** axillofemoral and **(B)** above-knee femoropopliteal sites.

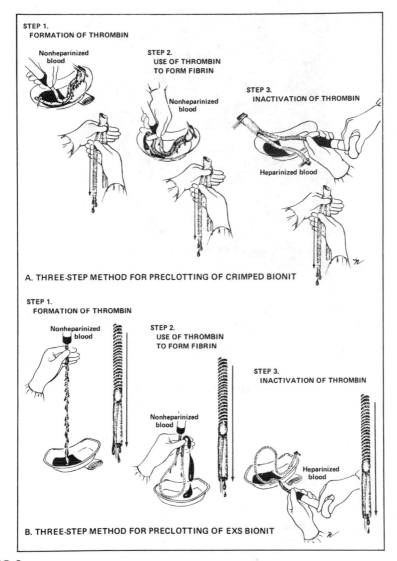

FIG 9.
Preclotting sequence for **(A)** crimped and **(B)** externally supported *(EXS)* knitted Dacron grafts.

ability to predict whether a dog would close a 4-mm diameter, 6-cm length Dacron graft implanted in the carotid arteries. She has been able to do this with almost 100% accuracy.[64] We are in the process now of carrying these experimental observations into clinical practice. It is my belief that the initial falloff we see in nearly all life tables before patency rates level off is due to the implantation of synthetic grafts in patients who would be better

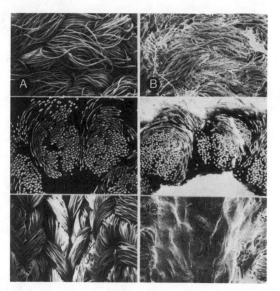

FIG 10.
Bionit II warp-knit, external-velour prosthesis before preclotting **(A)** and after pre-clotting **(B).** *Top,* scanning electron microscopy (SEM) of outer surfaces. *Middle,* light microscopy of longitudinal sections with flow surfaces at bottom. Hematoxy-lin-eosin stain of specimen on right. *Bottom,* SEM of inner surfaces. Approximate original magnifications, ×50. (From Sauvage LR, Davis CC, Smith JC, et al: Development and clinical use of porous Dacron arterial prostheses, in Sawyer PN [ed]: *Modern Vascular Grafts.* New York, McGraw-Hill Book Co, 1987, p 244. Used by permission.)

served by grafts with endothelial surfaces. If we could identify before surgery the patients with high thrombotic potential who really need grafts with endothelial surfaces, we should obtain primary above-knee femoropopliteal graft patencies at 5 years in the 90% rather than 60% to 70% range for an aggregate of patients with a wide spread of thrombotic potentials. I further believe that, with the development of appropriate antithrombotic agents for enhancing prostacyclin secretion while depressing thromboxane formation, if we must use prostheses for patients with high thrombotic potential we will be able to convert them biochemically to a lower thrombotic potential and obtain high patency rates for them also. There is much room for progress in this area. We now know that there are different subsets of dogs in the experimental laboratory and we screen them for use in our studies according to their thrombotic potential.[65] In other words, if we want a rigorous test of a pharmacologic agent or a new graft in the carotid artery, we will implant the graft in animals that have a high thrombotic potential that would rapidly close an ordinary graft or one unprotected by pharmaoclogic means. We do not have to implant nearly as many grafts when we perform our studies in this manner, and we obtain

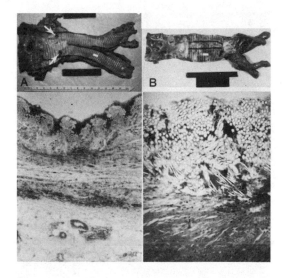

FIG 11.
A, Bionit II warp-knit external-velour aortic bifurcation explant with bilateral renal grafts. This graft was implanted 8 weeks before the patient, a 72-year-old man, died of renal failure. Arrows on the gross specimen indicate open orifices of renal artery grafts. The rectangle marks the area from which a specimen was taken for the light microscopy (LM) shown below (flow surface is at top). Tissue ingrowth extends into outer wall; flow surface is composed of compacted fibrin. Hematoxylin-eosin; approximate original magnification, ×40. **B,** Bionit II warp-knit external-velour aortic bifurcation explant. This graft was implanted 21 months before the patient, a 73-year-old man, died on the third day following aortocoronary bypass surgery. The rectangle marks the area from which the specimen was taken for the LM shown below (flow surface is at top). Tissue ingrowth extends into the outer wall; the flow surface is composed of a thin layer of fibrin. Hematoxylin-eosin; approximate original magnification, ×100. (Part A from Sauvage LR, Davis CC, Smith JC, et al: Development and clinical use of porous Dacron arterial prostheses, in Sawyer PN [ed]: *Modern Vascular Grafts*. New York, McGraw-Hill Book Co, 1987, p 231. Used by permission.)

information of greater validity more rapidly by categorizing our animals before involving them in given experiments. I suspect that information of this type will also prove to be very useful in the proper treatment of patients.

A recent experimental development in our laboratory has been an improved method for formation of an impervious knitted graft in manufacture by the hydraulic impaction of a glutaraldehyde-albumin matrix (Fig 12). These grafts have zero porosity at 120 mm Hg. They have good surgical handling characteristics and heal reasonably well in the canine descending thoracic aorta but not as well as a properly preclotted graft. However, we have observed that the albumin matrix has healed at least as well as the preclotted graft in the carotid-femoral position in the dog.

The necessity to preclot is an inconvenience in the use of knitted grafts,

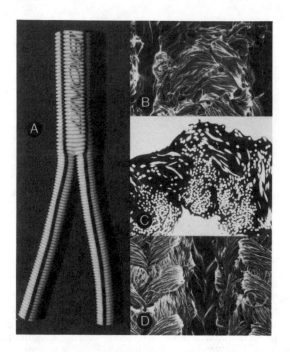

FIG 12.
A, Bionit bifurcation graft with albumin matrix. **B,** scanning electron microscopy (SEM) of external surface. **C,** light microscopy of longitudinal section with flow surface at bottom. Hemtoxylin-eosin. **D,** SEM of internal surface. Approximate original magnifications, ×50.

and for this reason woven grafts are popular for use in the aortoiliac area despite poor surgical handling and healing characteristics. I believe that grafts made impervious in manufacture by the impaction of a biologic compound will come to have significant clinical use in the next several years.

Arterial Patches

Patch graft angioplasty is very important in my clinical practice; I use a Dacron patch in perhaps one in five or six carotid endarterectomies and quite frequently in peripheral artery reconstructions of one type or another (Fig 13). My first use of patch grafts involved simply opening a crimped graft and fashioning a patch from it, and these worked satisfactorily. However, as mentioned previously, we subsequently developed a specific fabric for intracardiac and arterial use.[42-44] This warp-knit double-velour Dacron patch discussed for intracardiac use also works very well for arterial patching. I believe that these grafts heal quite rapidly by pannus ingrowth from the edge, as well as transinterstices ingrowth from the perigraft tissue response. Healing is a function of the patch graft's width, not its length. In

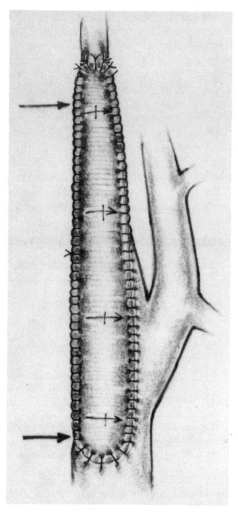

FIG 13.
Dacron patch angioplasty of the carotid. If fabric is positioned as illustrated by arrows, a desirable, but not excessive, doming effect will be achieved. (From Schultz GA, Zammit M, Sauvage LR, et al: Carotid artery Dacron patch graft angioplasty: A ten-year experience. *J Vasc Surg* 1987; 5:476. Used by permission.)

essence, it represents the healing of a wide, linear anastomosis. A 10-mm wide patch requires only 5-mm pannus ingrowth from each side to reach the middle and completely resurface it with true vascular healing.

So much for the past. What of the next 5 years? I offer these predictions:

1. The St. Jude valve will continue to be the prosthesis of choice for most patients in whom low-dose anticoagulation is not contraindicated.

2. The bioprosthetic porcine valves will continue to be the prostheses of choice for most patients over 75 years old in normal sinus rhythm who require aortic valve replacement. Cryopreserved homograft valves appear to be superior, but lack of availability will limit their application.

3. Diagnostic tests will be developed to enable the thrombotic potential of patients to be rapidly determined so that the proper graft type can be selected. I see this as a needed advance of the greatest importance.

4. Porous grafts will be developed that can be rendered impervious by a single exposure to whole blood, enabling biosynthetic composite prostheses of fibrin and Dacron to gain wider usage.

5. Knitted Dacron grafts will be manufactured with an impervious protein matrix with chemical constituents that will make the flow surface hypothrombogenic and the outer surface highly conducive to healing, enabling one composite prosthesis to be used from the ascending aorta to the above-knee popliteal.

6. The saphenous autograft will continue to be the conduit of choice for below-knee bypass.

References

1. Sauvage LR, Wood SJ: Technique for correction of mitral insufficiency by leaflet advancement. *J Thorac Cardiovasc Surg* 1966; 51:649–655.
2. Starr A, Edwards ML: Mitral replacement: Clinical experience with a ball-valve prosthesis. *Ann Surg* 1961; 154:726–740.
3. Cobanoglu A, Fessler CL, Guvendik L, et al: Aortic valve replacement with the Starr-Edwards prosthesis: A comparison of the first and second decades of follow-up. *Ann Thorac Surg* 1988; 45:248–252.
4. Sauvage LR, Wood SJ: Prosthesis development, in Sauvage LR, Viggers RF, Berger K, et al (eds): *Prosthetic Replacement of the Aortic Valve.* Springfield, Ill, Charles C Thomas Publisher, 1972, p 181.
5. Sauvage LR, Wood SJ, Berger KE: Prosthetic aortic valve replacement: An experimental study in the calf. *Surgery* 1965; 57:175–183.
6. Sauvage LR, Viggers RF, Berger K, et al: Aortic ball valve design based upon healing and hydraulic considerations. *Surgery* 1970; 67:151–167.
7. Sauvage LR, Wood SJ: Prosthesis development, in Sauvage LR, Viggers RF, Berger K, et al (eds): *Prosthetic Replacement of the Aortic Valve.* Springfield, Ill, Charles C Thomas Publisher, 1972, p 189.
8. Viggers RF, Robel SB, Wood SJ, et al: Improvement of aortic ball valve function by flow guidance. *Surgery* 1968; 63:52–58.
9. Sauvage LR, Berger K, Wood SJ: The clinical significance of healing data obtained from the study of prosthetic valves in animals. *Adv Cardiol* 1972; 7:25–33.
10. Sauvage LR, Berger KE, Wood SJ, et al: Influence of amount of exposed fabric on thrombotic complications of aortic ball valves in the calf. *Am J Surg* 1968; 116:260–265.
11. Berger K: Healing of the encapsulable parts of aortic valve prostheses, in Sauvage LR, Viggers RF, Berger K, et al (eds): *Prosthetic Replacement of the Aortic Valve.* Springfield, Ill, Charles C Thomas Publisher, 1972, pp 81–118.
12. Björk VO, Henze A, Holmgren A: Five years' experience with the Björk-Shiley

tilting-disc valve in isolated aortic valvular disease. *J Thorac Cardiovasc Surg* 1974; 68:393–404.

13. Björk VO, Henze A: Ten years' experience with the Björk-Shiley tilting-disc valve. *J Thorac Cardiovasc Surg* 1979; 78:331–342.

14. Flemma RJ, Mullen DC, Kleinman LH, et al: Survival and "event-free" analysis of 785 patients with Björk-Shiley spherical-disc valves at 10 to 16 years. *Ann Thorac Surg* 1988; 45:258–272.

15. Lindblom D: Long-term results after aortic valve replacement with the Björk-Shiley prosthesis. *J Thorac Cardiovasc Surg* 1988; 95:658–667.

16. Emery RW, Mettler E, Nicoloff DM: A new cardiac prosthesis: The St. Jude Medical cardiac valve. *Circulation* 1979; 60(suppl 1):I48–I54.

17. Chaux A, Gray RJ, Matloff JM, et al: An appreciation of the new St. Jude valvular prosthesis. *J Thorac Cardiovasc Surg* 1981; 81:202–211.

18. Debakey ME: *Advances in Cardiac Valves: Clinical Perspectives.* New York, Yorke Medical Books, 1983, pp 14–24, 108–114.

19. Chaux A, Czer LSC, Matloff JM, et al: The St. Jude Medical bileaflet valve prosthesis: A 5-year experience. *J Thorac Cardiovasc Surg* 1984; 88:706–717.

20. Arom KV, Nicoloff DM, Kersten TE, et al: Six years of experience with the St. Jude Medical valvular prosthesis. *Circulation* 1985; 72(suppl 2):II153–II158.

21. Baudet EM, Oca CC, Roques XF, et al: A 5-½ year experience with the St. Jude Medical cardiac valve prosthesis. *J Thorac Cardiovasc Surg* 1985; 90:137–144.

22. Duncan JM, Cooley DA, Reul GJ, et al: Durability and low thrombogenicity of the St. Jude Medical valve at 5-year follow-up. *Ann Thorac Surg* 1986; 42:500–505.

23. Czer LSC, Matloff JM, Chaux A, et al: The St. Jude valve: Analysis of thromboembolism, warfarin-related hemorrhage, and survival. *Am Heart J* 1987; 114:389–397.

24. Kopf GS, Hammond GL, Geha AS, et al: Long-term performance of the St. Jude Medical valve: Low incidence of thromboembolism and hemorrhagic complications with modest doses of warfarin. *Circulation* 1987; 76(suppl 3):III132–III136.

25. Buch WS, Kosek JC, Angell WW: Deterioration of formalin-treated aortic valve heterografts. *J Thorac Cardiovasc Surg* 1970; 60:673–682.

26. Horowitz MS, Goodman D, Fogarty TJ, et al: Mitral valve replacement with the glutaraldehyde-preserved porcine heterograft. *J Thorac Cardiovasc Surg* 1974; 67:885–895.

27. Davila JC, Magilligan DJ Jr: Experience with the Hancock porcine xenograft for mitral replacement, in Davila JC (ed): *Second Henry Ford Hospital International Symposium on Cardiac Surgery.* New York, Appleton-Century-Crofts, 1977, pp 485–490.

28. Oyer PE, Stinson EB, Reitz BA, et al: Long-term evaluation of the porcine xenograft bioprosthesis. *J Thorac Cardiovasc Surg* 1979; 78:343–350.

29. Gallo I, Ruiz B, Duran CMG: Five- to 8-year follow-up of patients with the Hancock cardiac bioprosthesis. *J Thorac Cardiovasc Surg* 1983; 86:897–902.

30. Carpentier A, Lemaigre G, Robert L, et al: Biological factors affecting long-term results of valvular heterografts. *J Thorac Cardiovasc Surg* 1969; 58:467–483.

31. Carpentier A, Deloche A, Relland J, et al: Six-year follow-up of glutaraldehyde-preserved heterografts with particular reference to the healing of congenital valve malformations. *J Thorac Cardiovasc Surg* 1974; 68:771–782.

32. Bloomfield P, Kitchen AH, Wheatley DJ, et al: A prospective evaluation of the Björk-Shiley, Hancock and Carpentier-Edwards heart valve prostheses. *Circulation* 1985; 73:1213–1222.
33. Hartz RS, Fisher EB, Finkelmeier B, et al: An 8-year experience with porcine bioprosthetic cardiac valves. *J Thorac Cardiovasc Surg* 1986; 91:910–917.
34. Spencer FC, Grossi EA, Culliford AT, et al: Experiences with 1,643 porcine prosthetic valves in 1,492 patients. *Ann Surg* 1986; 203:691–700.
35. Hammond GL, Geha AS, Kopf GS, et al: Biological versus mechanical valves: Analysis of 1,116 valves inserted in 1,012 adult patients with a 4,818 patient-year and a 5,327 valve-year follow-up. *J Thorac Cardiovasc Surg* 1987; 93:182–198.
36. Nashef SAM, Sethia B, Turner MA, et al: Björk-Shiley and Carpentier-Edwards valves. *J Thorac Cardiovasc Surg* 1987; 93:394–404.
37. Berger K, Sauvage LR, Wood SJ, et al: Sewing ring healing of cardiac valve prostheses. *Surgery* 1967; 61:102–117.
38. Sauvage LR, Viggers RF, Berger K, et al: Aortic ball valve design based upon healing and hydraulic considerations. *Surgery* 1970; 67:151–167.
39. Sauvage LR, Wood SJ: Prosthesis development, in Sauvage LR, Viggers RF, Berger K, et al (eds): *Prosthetic Replacement of the Aortic Valve*. Springfield, Ill, Charles C Thomas Publisher, 1972, p 194.
40. Sauvage LR: Prosthetic valves 1977: A retrospective analysis and a look to the future. *Med Instrum* 1977; 11:107–109.
41. Hirsh J, Levine MN: The optimal intensity of oral anticoagulant therapy. *JAMA* 1987; 258:2723–2726.
42. Barros D'Sa AAB, Berger K, Di Benedetto G, et al: A healable filamentous Dacron surgical fabric: Experimental studies and clinical experience. *Ann Surg* 1980; 192:645–657.
43. Schultz GA, Zammit M, Sauvage LR, et al: Carotid artery Dacron patch graft angioplasty: A ten-year experience. *J Vasc Surg* 1987; 5:475–478.
44. Carney WI Jr, Lilly MP: Intraoperative evaluation of PTFE, Dacron and autogenous vein as carotid patch materials. *Ann Vasc Surg* 1987; 1:583–586.
45. DeBakey ME, Jordan GL Jr, Abbott JP, et al: Fate of Dacron vascular grafts. *Arch Surg* 1964; 89:757–782.
46. Wesolowski SA, Fries CC, McMahon JD, et al: A new vascular prosthesis: Preliminary report. *Trans Am Soc Artif Intern Organs* 1965; 11:330–335.
47. Berger K, Sauvage LR: Late fiber deterioration in Dacron arterial grafts. *Ann Surg* 1981; 193:477–491.
48. Sauvage LR, Berger K, Wood SJ, et al: A very thin, porous, knitted arterial prosthesis: Experimental data and early clinical assessment. *Surgery* 1969; 65:78–88.
49. Berger K, Sauvage LR, Rao AM, et al: Healing of arterial prostheses in man: Its incompleteness. *Ann Surg* 1972; 175:118–127.
50. Wesolowski SA, Sauvage LR, Golaski WM, et al: Rationale for the development of the gossamer small arterial prosthesis. *Arch Surg* 1968; 97:864–871.
51. Sauvage LR, Berger KE, Mansfield PB, et al: Future directions in the development of arterial prostheses for small and medium caliber arteries. *Surg Clin North Am* 1974; 54:213–228.
52. Sauvage LR, Berger K, Wood SJ, et al: An external velour surface for porous arterial prostheses. *Surgery* 1971; 70:940–953.
53. Wu H-D, Zammit M, Sauvage LR, et al: The influence of inner wall filamentousness on the performance of small- and large-caliber arterial grafts. *J Vasc Surg* 1985; 2:255–262.

54. Yates SG, Barros D'Sa AAB, Berger K, et al: The preclotting of porous arterial prostheses. *Ann Surg* 1978; 188:611–622.
55. Sauvage LR, Berger K, Wood SJ, et al: The USCI-Sauvage filamentous vascular prosthesis: Rationale, clinical results, and healing in man, in Sawyer PN, Kaplitt MJ (eds): *Vascular Grafts*. New York, Appleton-Century-Crofts, 1977, pp 185–196.
56. Mathisen SR, Wu H-D, Sauvage LR, et al: The influence of denier and porosity on performance of a warp-knit Dacron arterial prosthesis. *Ann Surg* 1986; 203:382–389.
57. Bethea MC, Reemtsma K: Graft hemostasis: An alternative to preclotting. *Ann Thorac Surg* 1979; 27:374.
58. Cooley DA, Romagnoli A, Milam JD, et al: A method of preparing woven Dacron aortic grafts to prevent interstitial hemorrhage. *Cardiovasc Dis Bull Texas Heart Inst* 1981; 8:49–51.
59. Rumisek JD, Wade CE, Brooks DE, et al: Heat-denatured albumin-coated Dacron vascular grafts: Physical characteristics and in vivo performance. *J Vasc Surg* 1986; 4:136–143.
60. Sauvage LR, Berger K, Barros D'Sa AAB, et al: Dacron arterial prostheses, in Dardik H (ed): *Graft Materials in Vascular Surgery*. Miami, Symposia Specialists Inc, 1978, pp 153–168.
61. Kenney DA, Sauvage LR, Wood SJ, et al: Comparison of noncrimped, externally supported (EXS) and crimped, nonsupported Dacron prostheses for axillofemoral and above-knee femoropopliteal bypass. *Surgery* 1982; 92:931–946.
62. Schultz GA, Sauvage LR, Mathisen SR, et al: A 5- to 7-year experience with externally supported Dacron prostheses in axillofemoral and femoropopliteal bypass. *Ann Vasc Surg* 1986; 1:214–224.
63. Kremen AF, Mendez-Fernandez MA, Geis RC, et al: The Dacron EXS graft: Patency in femoropopliteal and femorotibial surgery. *J Cardiovasc Surg* 1986; 27:125–130.
64. Zammit M, Kaplan S, Sauvage LR, et al: Aspirin therapy in small-caliber arterial prostheses: Long-term experimental observations. *J Vasc Surg* 1984; 1:839–851.
65. Kaplan S, Marcoe KF, Sauvage LR, et al: The effect of predetermined thrombotic potential of the recipient on small-caliber graft performance. *J Vasc Surg* 1986; 3:311–321.

Intraoperative Echocardiography: A Practical Approach

Bruce P. Mindich, M.D.

Division of Cardiovascular Surgery, St. Luke's/Roosevelt Hospital Center,
New York, New York

Martin E. Goldman, M.D.

Division of Cardiology, Mt. Sinai School of Medicine, New York, New York

Intraoperative echocardiography, which images the cardiac chambers and valves in real time, has become the standard technique for evaluating ventricular and valvular function in the operating room.[1] Intraoperative echocardiography offers significant advantages over the routine nonphysiologic techniques for evaluation of ventricular and valve function, particularly digital palpation, insufflation, hemodynamic measurements, and dye dilution curves. Recently, color-flow Doppler has been applied intraoperatively to image blood flow within the cardiac chambers.[2] This chapter will focus on the practical applications of intraoperative echocardiography for evaluating valvular and ventricular function.

Definitions

M-mode echocardiography is a noninvasive imaging technique that emits a single, thin ultrasound beam from a transducer, which travels in a straight line, reflecting off the cardiac structures in its path and returning to the transducer. The M-mode display demonstrates the motion of the cardiac structures along that single beam over time. *Two-dimensional (2-D) echocardiography* is a multibeam interrogation of a larger sector of the heart that provides information regarding density and location of cardiac structures. The images are seen in real time and stored on a video cassette tape (Fig 1). *Doppler echocardiography* evaluates blood flow velocity by emitting sound waves at a known frequency directed at a moving sample volume of blood. The sound wave frequency is altered or shifted, depending upon the velocity and direction of the blood (the Doppler shift), which is depicted by an audio signal and a spectral display. Routine *pulsed Doppler* samples Doppler shift information from blood flow at a particular site along a single ultrasound beam (Fig 2). *Continuous-wave* Doppler

Adv Card Surg 1:223–248, 1990
© 1990, Year Book Medical Publishers, Inc.
0889-5074/90/01-223-248-$04.00

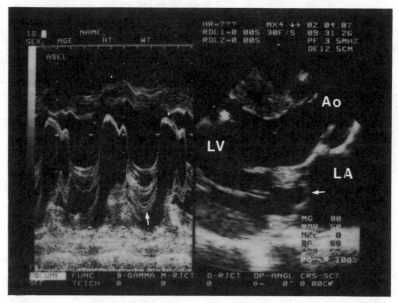

FIG 1.
Intraoperative two-dimensional (2-D) and M-mode echo. The 2-D echo **(right)** is a systolic. long-axis view demonstrating dramatic prolapse of the posterior mitral valve leaflet *(arrow)*. M-mode **(left)** is obtained by imaging through a single ultrasound beam at the mitral valve level. The mitral valve, which is seen through three diastolic periods (M-shaped), demonstrates holosystolic prolapse *(arrow)*. Ao = aorta; *LA* = left atrium; *LV* = left ventricle.

samples and receives blood flow information along the entire beam of the sound wave. Pulsed Doppler interrogates specific sites along the emitted beam (i.e., for localizing source and extent of mitral regurgitation or differentiating ventricular septal defect from mitral regurgitation), while continuous-wave Doppler is applied to resolve higher velocities (i.e., aortic stenosis; Fig 3). *Color-flow* (real-time) Doppler displays Doppler shift information over a wide sector of blood flow in different colors (depending on blood flow direction, velocity, and turbulence) superimposed over the 2-D anatomic image. *Contrast 2-D echocardiography* involves injection of sterile saline or dextrose water into a cardiac chamber, creating echogenic microbubbles or "contrast." Microbubble movement is normally antegrade with blood flow but refluxes retrograde in valvular regurgitation.

There are two major modes of intraoperative echocardiography: *epicardial* and *transesophageal* 2-D echocardiography (Fig 4). Epicardial echocardiography is performed by a surgeon placing the sterilely prepared ultrasound transducer directly on the exposed epicardium. A degree of expertise in manipulation of the transducer, recognition of the image planes, and an assistant to adjust the machine are necessary to acquire an acceptable image. Intraoperative transesophageal echocardiography is usually the

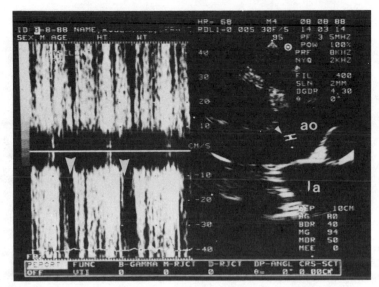

FIG 2.
Pulsed Doppler echo, aortic regurgitation. Two-dimensional echo **(right)** long-axis view, with pulsed Doppler sample volume marker *(arrowhead)* positioned in the left ventricular outflow tract. Pulsed Doppler spectral display **(left)** demonstrates diastolic turbulent flow *(between arrowheads)*. la = left atrium; ao = aorta.

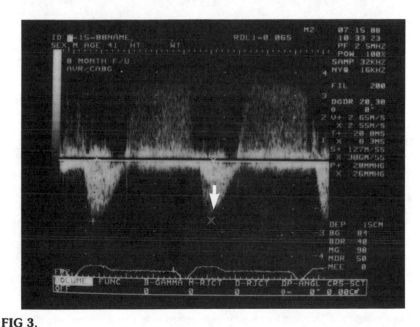

FIG 3.
Continuous-wave Doppler showing aortic stenosis and regurgitation. Blood flow moving away from transducer during systole is below the line *(arrow);* regurgitant flow is above the line.

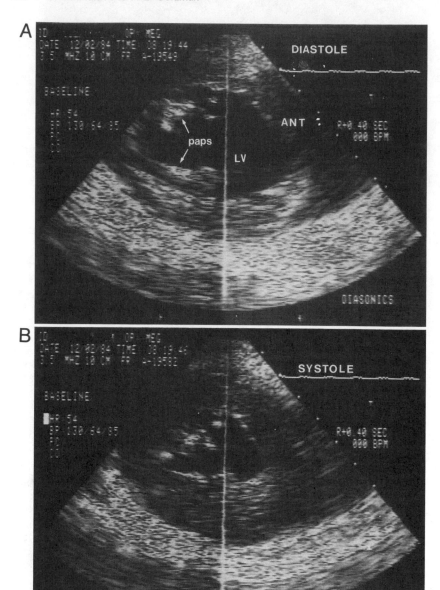

FIG 4.
Transesophageal echo: short axis, midpapillary muscle plane *(paps)*. **A,** diastolic frame: since heart is viewed from behind, the orientation is different than epicardial echo. *ANT* = anterior wall; *LV* = left ventricle. **B,** systolic frame: note uniform ventricular wall thickening.

domain of the anesthesiologist.[3-5] A small ultrasonic transducer is fixed to the end of a gastroscope and introduced via the esophagus into a retrocardiac position, yielding several planes for evaluation of the heart. With transesophageal echo, imaging can be done continuously throughout the operative procedure without necessitating direct manipulation of the transducer on the heart (Table 1).

Practical Applications

Similar views are obtainable by either epicardial or transesophageal echocardiography. The major distinction is that transesophageal echocardiography images the heart from a retrocardiac position, and therefore the orientation is a mirror image of the epicardial "antecardiac" position. Since epicardial echocardiography is the technique most often used by surgeons, we will focus on that application for this chapter.

Any ultrasound machine and transducer can be utilized for intraoperative imaging if properly prepared. Since gas or liquid sterilization may interfere with normal functioning of delicate ultrasonic equipment, the transducer can be covered with a sterile sheath from its tip down the length of its cord to avoid contamination (Fig 5). Following sternotomy and pericardiotomy, the sterilely prepared transducer is then placed directly on the exposed epicardium to gain initial orientation. The pericardial space can be filled with saline to provide an interface between the transducer and the epicardium. Alternatively, sterile acoustic gel can be placed on the inside of the sterile drape covering the transducer. The echocardiographer must not apply excessive pressure with the transducer on the epicardium; otherwise, the cardiac chambers will be distorted. Proper technique may be facilitated

TABLE 1.
Comparison of Epicardial With Transesophageal Intraoperative Echocardiography

Variable	Epicardial	Transesophageal
Transducer	Hand-held	Gastroscope mounted
Anatomic orientation	Anteroposterior	Posteroanterior
Equipment	Any	Specialized transducer
Views	All except apex	All including apex
Imaging	Intermittent	Continuous
Advantages	Rapid manipulation	Applicable for noncardiac surgery or intensive care unit postoperatively

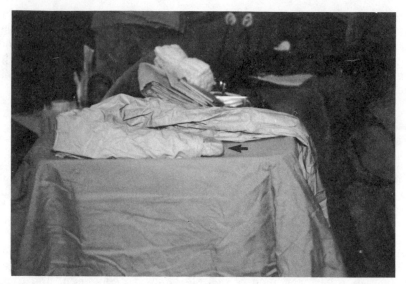

FIG 5.
Transducer sterile preparation. The head of the probe is enclosed in a clear sterile drape with gel *(arrow)*. The cord is covered with a blue nonabsorbable orthopedic sleeve.

by resting the wrist on the sternal retractor, thereby leaving the hand flexible at the wrist to move with the cardiac motion.

Several routine views are obtainable by epicardial echocardiography (Table 2). In the long axis view, one can see the mitral valve opening in diastole and closing in systole, the left atrium, aortic valve, parts of the interventricular septum, and posterior wall (see Fig 1). If the transducer is then rotated 90° in a clockwise or counterclockwise rotation, the short axis view of the heart can be obtained, providing circumferential slices of the heart. If the transducer is arced toward the great vessels, the aorta, left atrium, and parts of the tricuspid valve are seen (Fig 6). If the transducer is arced gradually toward the apex, the mitral valve in the short axis can be seen opening and closing (Fig 7). Circumferential ventricular function at the midpapillary muscle level can be imaged by pointing the transducer more apically (Fig 8). By returning the transducer to the long axis view and rotating it and arcing slightly medially, the right ventricular inflow view is seen, with the anterior and septal leaflets of the tricuspid valve and parts of the right ventricle and right atrium (Fig 9). If the transducer is rotated clockwise and arced slightly superiorly from the long axis view, the pulmonic valve and bifurcation of the pulmonary artery are seen. The transducer can also be placed on the great vessels to evaluate the aortic root, the ascending aorta, and the bifurcation of the pulmonary artery. The true apex of the ventricle cannot be adequately visualized by epicardial echo without distortion of the heart.

TABLE 2.
Intraoperative 2-D Echo Planes and Their
Application

Long axis (see Fig 1)
   Mitral stenosis: doming, calcified valve
   Mitral regurgitation: pathology, quantify regurgitation
   Aortic stenosis: assess valve excursion
   Aortic regurgitation: quantify regurgitation
   Left ventricular function
Short axis: aorta/left atrium (see Fig 6)
   Aortic cusps
   Left atrial size
   Localized mitral regurgitation jet in left atrium
   Localizing aortic regurgitation jet
   Pulmonary artery
Short axis: mitral valve level (see Fig 7)
   Anterior and posterior leaflets
   Mitral anulus
   Mitral regurgitant jet
   Aortic regurgitant jet over anterior leaflet of mitral valve
Short axis: papillary muscle (see Fig 8)
   Circumferential slice of left ventricle
   Left ventricle muscle function
   Left ventricle muscle thickness
   Hypertrophic myopathy
   Local contractile abnormalities
Right ventricular inflow: tricuspid valve (see Fig 9)
   Tricuspid regurgitation
Aortic root
   Aortic velocity
   Aortic dissection

Transesophageal echocardiography can obtain planes similar to those imaged by epicardial echocardiography. Additionally, from the base of the heart pointing apically, a foreshortened four-chamber view can also be visualized. The transesophageal view can also detect the left atrial appendage and may be more sensitive for detection of mitral regurgitation than epicardial echo.

Evaluation of Mitral Regurgitation

Mitral regurgitation can be due to primary valvular disease such as mitral valve prolapse, ruptured chordae, flail leaflets, or endocarditis or secondary to myocardial disease such as papillary muscle dysfunction, left ventric-

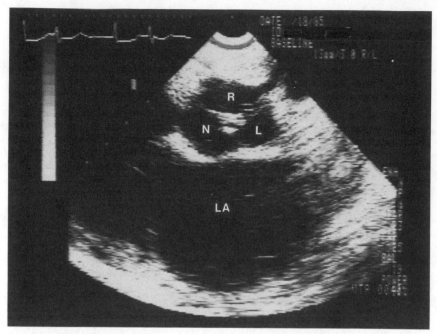

FIG 6.
Short-axis view, aortic level. *LA* = left atrium. Three coronary cusps: *L* = left; *N* = noncoronary; *R* = right.

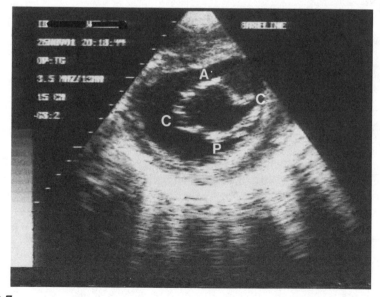

FIG 7.
Short-axis view, mitral valve level. *A* = anterior leaflet; *C* = commissures; *P* = posterior leaflet.

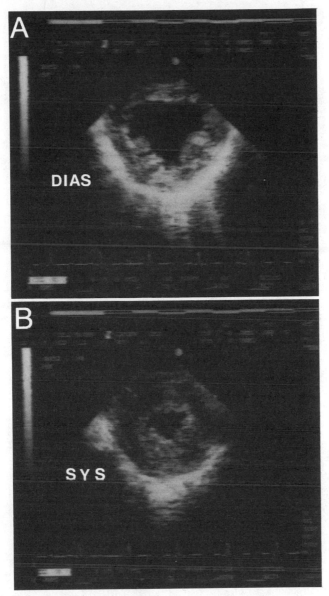

FIG 8.
Short axis, papillary muscle level. **A,** diastolic frame. **B,** systolic frame.

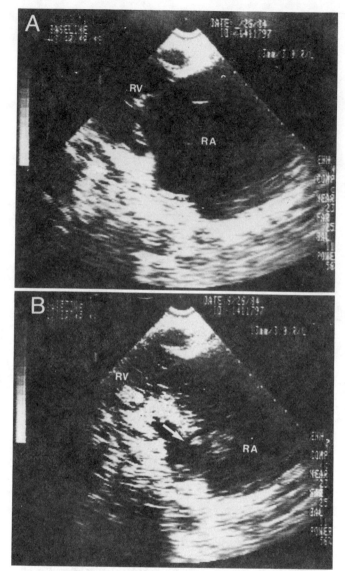

FIG 9.
Tricuspid regurgitation, contrast, **A,** right ventricular *(RV)* inflow view: giant right atrium *(RA)* is imaged. **B,** contrast injection: systolic jet of tricuspid regurgitation *(arrow)* refluxing into RA.

ular dilatation, and ischemic heart disease. The valvular anatomy can be imaged just before the operative procedure by either transesophageal or epicardial echocardiography to better define the pathology and to determine whether valve repair is feasible. If the etiology of the mitral regurgitation is rheumatic heart disease, intraoperative echo can accurately detect the extent of subvalvular calcification and fibrosis, which may affect the decision to repair or replace the valve. Ruptured chordae or flail anterior leaflet may negate reparative efforts. Additionally, the relative severity of mitral regurgitation can be detected by either contrast echocardiography or color-flow Doppler.

Contrast echocardiography for detection of mitral regurgitation is performed by passing a needle through the right ventricle and interventricular septum and into the left ventricle, through which hand-agitated sterile fluid is injected (5% dextrose in water [D5W], normal saline, or a mixture of sterile fluid with blood) rapidly (avoiding ventricular premature beats). Location of the transseptal needle can be ascertained either by 2-D echo or by hemodynamic monitoring through a three-way stopcock. This injection generates microbubbles (ranging from 5 to 120 μm in size), which normally fill the left ventricle completely and exit antegrade out of the aorta during one to two systolic contractions; however, if there is mitral regurgitation, reflux into the left atrium will occur with each systolic contraction[6, 7] (Fig 10). The severity of regurgitation can be assessed based on the relative density of microbubbles filling the left atrium and the time for their complete clearing from the left atrium. In a study by Goldman et al.,[8] there was an excellent correlation between intraoperative contrast echocardiography and cardiac catheterization for the detection of mitral regurgitation (100% sensitivity, 97% specificity in 120 cases). More importantly, there was a .93 correlation between the quantification of the severity of mitral regurgitation determined preoperatively by cardiac catheterization and that determined by intraoperative contrast echocardiography in 120 patients.

Color-flow echocardiography can also detect the presence or absence of mitral regurgitation. Color-Doppler echocardiography detects blood flow velocity (from the Doppler shift) over a wide anatomic sector, displayed by distinctive color patterns. The colors represent the direction (red hues encoding blood moving toward, blue for blood moving away from the transducer), relative velocity (blood moving at higher velocities in lighter shades), and turbulence (blood flow moving in a random, rapid fashion is presented in a yellow, cyan, or mosaic pattern). The color-flow examination can monitor every heartbeat without injection of microbubbles. Laminar blood flow moving antegrade out the ventricle in systole would be depicted in a solid color and turbulent blood flow refluxing into the left atrium would appear as a mosaic color. The relative severity of mitral regurgitation is based on the relative size of the regurgitant mosaic-colored area filling the left atrium in both the long and short axis plane (Fig 11). As in contrast echocardiography, both the long and short axes are imaged to obtain a stereoscopic impression of the relative severity of regurgitation as well as to localize the precise source of the regurgitation.[2] Since the blood

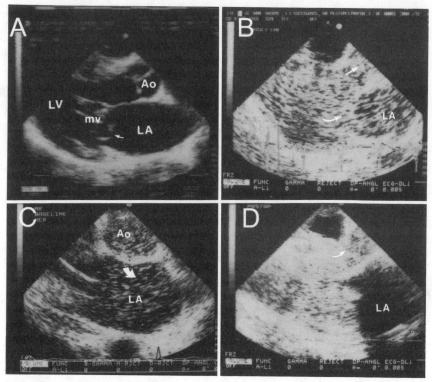

FIG 10.
Two-dimensional contrast echo: mitral regurgitation (MR). **A,** baseline long-axis view: flail posterior mitral leaflet *(arrow)* fails to coapt. Ao = aorta; LA = left atrium; LV = left ventricle; mv = mitral valve. **B,** contrast injection, long axis. Rapid injection of agitated saline introduces thousands of microbubbles into the LV, some exiting antegrade out the Ao *(straight arrow),* some refluxing retrograde into the LA *(curved arrow),* consistent with severe MR. **C,** contrast injection, short axis. Microbubbles fill the LA *(arrow)* and exit out the Ao. **D,** contrast injection, long axis. After procedure: following mitral repair, all microbubbles exit antegrade *(arrow),* none refluxing into the LA, confirming an adequate repair.

flow plane may be different than the anatomic plane, the surgeon is required to perform an intensive interrogation in multiple imaging planes to align the transducer into the proper flow plane. If the surgeon is not meticulous in the color-flow Doppler examination, the severity of regurgitation may be underestimated.[9] Calcified valves, aortic root or mitral anular calcification, and metallic surfaces of prosthetic valves may generate ultrasound artifacts, further complicating the Doppler examination (Fig 12, Table 3).

Since mechanical valve prostheses have potential thromboembolic and hemorrhagic complications, mitral valve repair offers an attractive alternative to valve replacement. Additionally, several studies have demonstrated

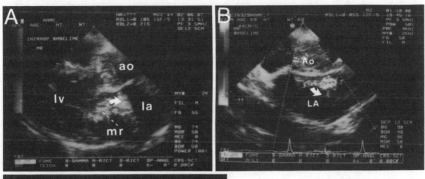

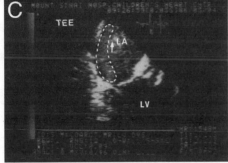

FIG 11.
Color Doppler: mitral regurgitation *(mr).* **A,** Long-axis view: systolic flow out of the aorta *(ao)* as well as turbulent flow retrograde into the left atrium *(la, arrow).* lv = left ventricle. **B,** short axis: the superior origin of the mr jet *(arrow)* is easily discerned. **C,** transesophageal echo *(TEE):* through modified basal two-chamber view, the mr jet *(encircled)* is seen extending deep into the LA.

that patients with mitral valve repair have better short- and long-term ventricular function compared with patients undergoing mitral valve replacement.[10, 11] Therefore, with echo/Doppler assistance, the surgeon can be more aggressive in his or her approach to valve repair surgery. Rapid physiologic evaluation of the repaired valve by intraoperative echo will determine if the valve repair is adequate. Either contrast or color Doppler can determine the presence and severity of regurgitation and localize its source immediately following cessation of cardiopulmonary bypass, while the patient is still cannulated. If more than minimal mitral regurgitation is present, the patient may require reinstitution of cardiopulmonary bypass for reexploration and repair.

Importantly, while the patient is coming off bypass, the echocardiogram can evaluate ventricular function. If the patient is hypotensive, a volume load or vasopressor may be necessary to raise systemic pressures to preoperative levels to evaluate the valve under physiologic circumstances. Even prosthetic valve dysfunction can be detected in the operating room, particularly if the valve is not seated properly or if retained chordae obstruct

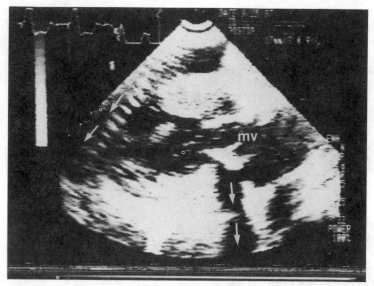

FIG 12.
Echo artifacts. Two different artifacts are depicted in this long-axis view: (1) mitral heterograft struts *(mv)* are echo-opaque and block transmission of ultrasound, creating echo-free areas behind them *(arrows)*; (2) artifact from a metallic instrument close to the transducer reverberates through the image *(arrows to the left)*.

valve closure. Additionally, in small ventricles with large hypertrophied walls, a larger mitral prosthesis (particularly the caged-ball type) may become dysfunctional due to the systolic contraction of the thick septum obstructing proper ball seating. This can be detected in the operating room while the patient is still cannulated, and the patient can then be placed on bypass again for reseating or replacing the prosthesis.

Tricuspid Regurgitation

Functional tricuspid regurgitation (TR) is usually secondary to pulmonary hypertension with subsequent right ventricular enlargement and anular dilatation. The presence of severe residual TR following mitral valve surgery increases the patient's morbidity and mortality significantly due to progressive right ventricular dysfunction. Unfortunately, routine physical examination and noninvasive or invasive evaluation may not accurately assess the severity of TR preoperatively. However, in a study by Goldman et al.,[12] intraoperative echocardiography was invaluable in determining which patients required tricuspid valve repair based on the presence of a markedly dilated tricuspid anulus and significant TR by contrast echocardiography. Both these findings suggest long-standing right ventricular dilatation; therefore, pulmonary pressures may remain elevated and fall slowly, and the anulus may remain dilated following mitral surgery, with resultant severe TR.

TABLE 3.
Comparison of Technique for Evaluation of Valvular Regurgitation

Variable	Contrast Echo	Color Echo
Equipment cost	$15,000	$100,000
Technical difficulty	Minimal	Difficult
Machine size	Small, large	Large
Observations	1–2 beats/injection	Every beat
Injections	+	−
Arrhythmogenic	+	−
False-positives	+ (VPB)*	+ (artifacts)
False-negatives	−	+ (angle dependent)
Noncardiac surgery	−	+ (transesophageal)

*VPB = ventricular premature beats; *plus sign* indicates present; *minus sign* indicates absent.

Conrast echocardiography of the tricuspid valve is performed by imaging the right ventricular inflow view and injecting microbubbles into the right ventricle, then determining the relative amount that refluxes retrograde into the right atrium (see Fig 9). Color Doppler can also be utilized to determine severity of tricuspid reflex (Fig 13). Ideally, the decision to repair the tricuspid valve should be made preoperatively; however, if intraoperative echocardiography is utilized, the amount of TR can be estimated intraoperatively before the mitral procedure. If there is severe TR, the tricuspid valve should be repaired immediately following the mitral procedure. However, if regurgitation is mild to moderate, it can be reassessed immediately following the mitral valve procedure while the patient is in sinus or paced rhythm following cessation of cardiopulmonary bypass. If there is significant residual pulmonary hypertension, dilated tricuspid anulus, and residual 3+ to 4+ TR, the tricuspid valve should be repaired.

Aortic Valve

Aortic regurgitation can also be evaluated with both contrast and color-flow echocardiography. For the evaluation of the aortic valve, contrast injections can be made either in the proximal aortic root or by fluid given through the aortic cannula. Retrograde flow into the left ventricle is indicative of the presence of aortic regurgitation. In 52 patients assessed by Goldman et al.,[8] the sensitivity was 91% and the specificity 100%, comparing intraoperative contrast echo with preoperative catheterization for determining the presence or absence of aortic regurgitation. Color Doppler can be used in a similar fashion (Fig 14).

Recently, surgeons have been more aggressive in aortic valve repair pro-

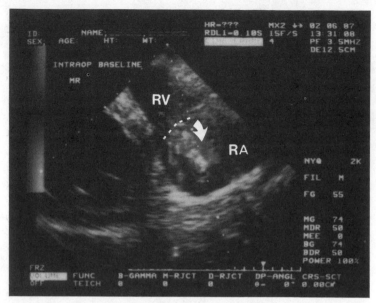

FIG 13.
Tricuspid regurgitation. The arrow depicts systolic reflux into the right atrium *(RA)*.
RV = right ventricle.

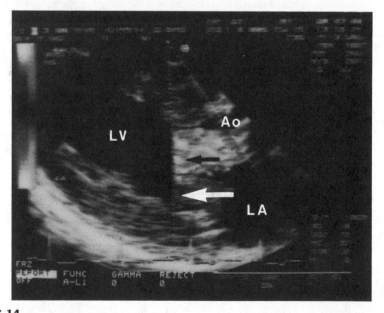

FIG 14.
Color long-axis view: normal mitral inflow *(white arrow)* is seen with severe aortic
(Ao) regurgitation *(black arrow)* filling the entire left ventricular *(LV)* outflow tract.
LA = left atrium.

cedures for calcific aortic stenosis, particularly with the introduction of ultrasonic debridement technology.[13] Intraoperative echocardiography can determine the mobility and relative severity of stenosis by imaging the aortic valve motion and excursion before a repair procedure is attempted (Fig 15). The severity of regurgitation can be assessed before and after the procedure as well. Continuous-wave Doppler performed by imaging from the ascending aorta can determine the peak and mean gradient across the aortic valve.

Combined Valvular Heart Disease

Intraoperative echocardiography may be particularly valuable when cardiac catheterization cannot assess the relative severity of the valve lesions. For instance, a patient who has significant aortic stenosis and mild to moderate mitral regurgitation may not require mitral surgery once the aortic obstruction is relieved. The severity of residual mitral regurgitation following the aortic operation is easily assessed with intraoperative echocardiography. If the patient is too ill to have a ventriculogram or aortogram before surgery, or if the patient is pregnant and radiation is to be avoided, intraoperative echo can assess both valvular and ventricular function.

Ventricular Function

Intraoperative echocardiography is invaluable for the on-line evaluation of ventricular function. By assessing the thickening of ventricular muscle and the relative cavity size, intraoperative echocardiography can detect changes in regional wall motion that may be secondary to acute myocardial ischemia or inadequate myocardial protection during bypass (Fig 16).[14-19]

Two-dimensional transesophageal echocardiography can detect myocardial ischemia manifested by wall motion and thickening (contraction) abnormalities before the development of ECG changes. Smith et al.,[20] using transesophageal echocardiography, found that 24 of 50 patients developed regional wall motion abnormalities consistent with intraoperative myocardial ischemia by transesophageal echocardiography, while only six of those episodes were detected by ECG monitoring. Therefore, intraoperative echo can rapidly detect ischemia and facilitate prompt therapeutic response to improve surgical outcome. By evaluating ventricular cavity size and contractility, the necessity for more or less volume or for myocardial inotropic agents can be determined objectively and instituted promptly. If a patient is hypotensive, intraoperative echo can evaluate ventricular chamber size and contractility to determine if the patient is hypovolemic or ischemic. A patient with ventricular hypertrophy may develop dynamic left ventricular outflow obstruction due to hypercontractility and hypovolemia[21] (Fig 17). The echocardiogram can determine ventricular function and volumes quickly to expedite appropriate therapeutic measures (volume infusion, β-blockers, or myomectomy).

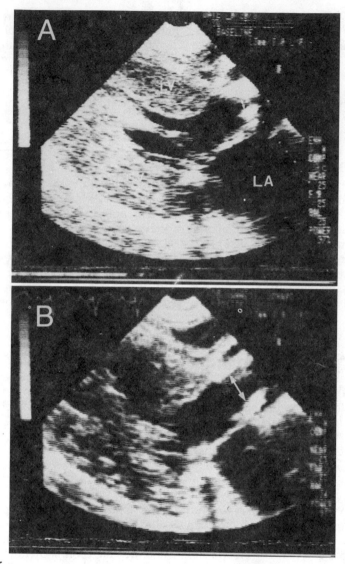

FIG 15.
Aortic stenosis. **A,** baseline: long-axis view demonstrates severely calcified aortic valve with markedly diminished systolic excursion *(arrows),* moderate concentric left ventricular *(LV)* hypertrophy, and a dilated left atrium *(LA).* **B,** following decalcification with high-frequency ultrasonic energy, the systolic excursion of the calcified leaflet is markedly improved.

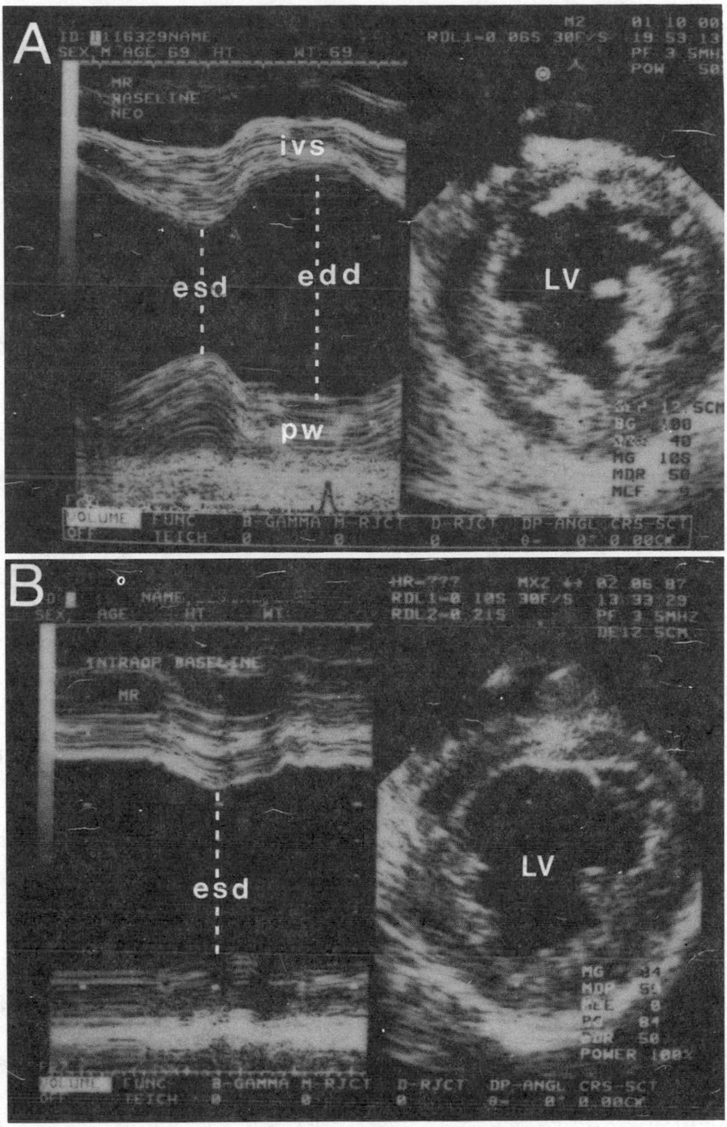

FIG 16.
Left ventricular *(LV)* function. **A,** M-mode *(left)* derived from the two-dimensional *(right)* view demonstrates normal systolic thickening and diastolic relaxation of the interventricular septum *(ivs)* and posterior wall *(pw)*, generating a smaller end-systolic cavity *(esd)* size than diastolic *(edd)*. **B,** a patient with inferoposterior infarction demonstrates no significant pw thickening.

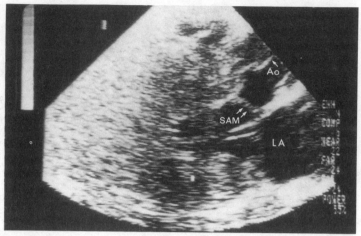

FIG 17.
Dynamic left ventricular outflow tract obstruction. Long-axis view demonstrating systolic anterior motion *(SAM)* of the anterior leaflet of the mitral valve *(two arrows)*, while the aortic *(Ao)* valve is open *(single arrow)*. LA = left atrium.

Coronary Arteries

High-frequency ultrasound transducers can image coronary arteries intra-operatively[22] (Fig 18). Hiratzka et al.[23] evaluated 82 coronary anastomoses for their patency and found a significant obstruction of an internal mammary to coronary artery anastomosis, which was then revised. Color Doppler could potentially evaluate flow through grafts and native coronary circulation. However, currently available instrumentation is technically too complex for routine clinical evaluation of coronary anatomy and flow.

Coronary Perfusion

An exciting new application of intraoperative echocardiography is in the evaluation of myocardial perfusion. We[24] reported the ability to determine the presence or absence of significant coronary lesions by using cardioplegic myocardial perfusion in a fashion similar to a thallium perfusion study. Using agitated saline or cardioplegic solution, perfusion could be determined in myocardial segments with adequate coronary flow; however, those muscle regions supplied by critical lesions had relative paucity of filling by contrast (Fig 19).

Congenital Heart Disease

Intraoperative echocardiography with either contrast or color Doppler can determine the presence of intracardiac or extracardiac shunt flow.[25-27]

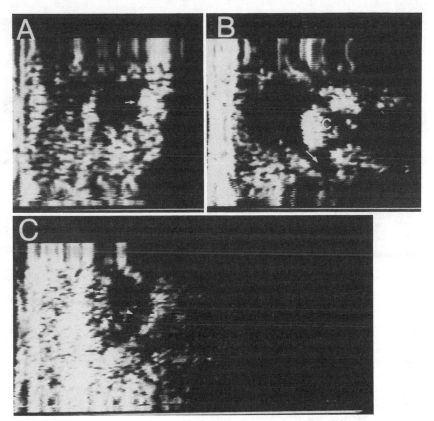

FIG 18.
High-frequency imaging of the coronary arteries. **A,** coronary artery: calcified plaque protrudes slightly into lumen *(arrow).* **B,** calcified plaque *(c)* at bifurcation *(arrow)* of coronary artery with shadowing artifact behind the calcium. **C,** diffuse thickening of the coronary lumen *(arrows).*

Ventricular septal defects may be multiple and may interdigitate through the septum. The entrance and exit through the septum can be easily detected using intracardiac imaging (Fig 20,A). Atrial septal defects can also be assessed rapidly using intraoperative echocardiography (Fig 20,B). Contrast injections or color-flow Doppler can be used to determine the shunt location. Postoperatively, before the patient is decannulated, the efficacy of the reparative surgical procedure can be rapidly assessed.

Intracardiac Tumors

Routine chest wall 2-D echocardiography, rapid computed tomography, and magnetic resonance imaging can noninvasively evaluate the presence

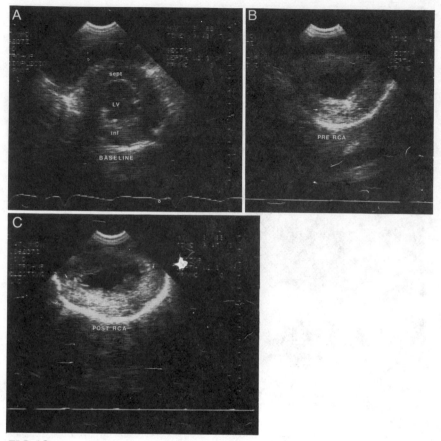

FIG 19.
Myocardial perfusion. **A,** baseline short-axis view, midpapillary muscle level. *inf* = inferior wall; *sept* = septum; *LV* = left ventricle. **B,** before coronary bypass, selective right coronary artery *(RCA)* injection delineating perfusion of limited myocardial segment *(arrows).* **C,** following distal anastomosis of right coronary graft and selective injection, contrast perfusion has much wider myocardial distribution *(arrows).*

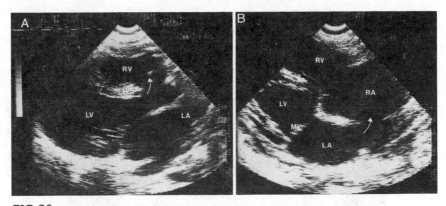

FIG 20.
Congenital heart disease. **A,** ventricular septal defect: long-axis view clearly demonstrates discontinuity of basal septum *(IVS)* consistent with large ventricular septal defect. *RV* = right ventricle; *LV* = left ventricle; *LA* = left atrium. **B,** atrial septal defect: modified RV inflow view angled to reveal four-chamber view depicts large atrial septal defect *(arrow)*. *RA* = right atrium; *MV* = mitral valve.

and extent of intracardiac malignant neoplasms.[28] Intraoperative echo can corroborate findings before the operative procedure (Fig 21). If extensive resection is required to remove the tumor, echo can assess ventricular and valvular function immediately before the patient leaves the operating room.

Aortic Dissection

Either epicardial echocardiography or transesophageal echocardiography can rapidly detect the origin of the intimal flap, which can facilitate the proper surgical approach to aortic dissection.[29, 30]

Summary

Intraoperative echocardiography is a reliable, rapid, and accurate technique to evaluate valvular and ventricular function that should facilitate therapeutic response and improve surgical outcome. Experience is required to obtain proper views and to interpret echocardiographic images. Though color-flow Doppler is more expensive and technically more complex than contrast echo, either technique can be utilized to evaluate valvular function. Utilizing intraoperative echo, surgeons can be more aggressive in reparative approaches to valvular lesions.

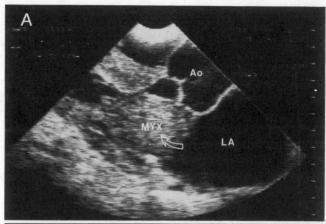

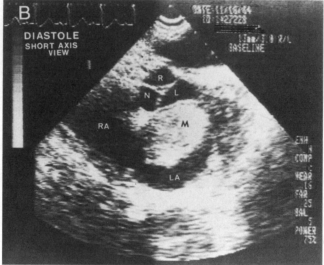

FIG 21.
Left atrial myxoma. **A,** long axis: the large tumor *(MYX)* enters the left ventricle, virtually occluding the mitral orifice *(arrow)*. Ao = aorta. **B,** short axis: myxoma *(M)*, its attachment to interatrial septum, and the three coronary cusps (right *[R]*, noncoronary *[N],* and left *[L]*) are seen. *RA* = right atrium; *LA* = left atrium.

References

1. Goldman ME, Mindich BP: Intraoperative two-dimensional echocardiography: New application of an old technique. *J Am Coll Cardiol* 1986; 7:374–382.
2. Czer LS, Maurer G, Bolger AF, et al: Intraoperative evaluation of mitral regurgitation by Doppler color flow mapping. *Circulation* 1987; 76:108–116.
3. Abel MD, Nishimura RA, Callahan MJ, et al: Evaluation of intraoperative

transesophageal two-dimensional echocardiography. *Anesthesiology* 1987; 66:64–68.

4. Thys DM, Hillel Z, Goldman ME, et al: A comparison of hemodynamic indices derived by invasive monitoring and two-dimensional echocardiography. *Anesthesiology* 1987; 67:630–634.

5. Konstadt SN, Thys D, Mindich BP, et al: Validation of quantitative intraoperative transesophageal echocardiography. *Anesthesiology* 1986; 65:418–421.

6. Goldman ME, Mindich BP, Teichholz LE, et al: Intraoperative contrast echocardiography to evaluate mitral valve operations. *J Am Coll Cardiol* 1984; 4:1035–1040.

7. Equaras MG, Pasalodos J, Gonzalez V, et al: Intraoperative contrast two-dimensional echocardiography: Evaluation of the presence and severity of aortic and mitral regurgitation during cardiac operations. *J Thorac Cardiovasc Surg* 1985; 89:573–579.

8. Goldman ME, Fuster V, Guarino T, et al: Intraoperative echocardiography for the evaluation of valvular regurgitation: Experience in 263 patients. *Circulation* 1986; 74:1143–1149.

9. Goldman ME, Mindich BP, Nanda NC: Intraoperative echocardiography: Who monitors the flood once the flood gates are opened? *J Am Coll Cardiol* 1988; 11:1362–1364.

10. Goldman ME, Mora F, Guarino T, et al: Mitral valvuloplasty is superior to valve replacement for preservation of left ventricular function: An intraoperative two-dimensional echocardiographic study. *J Am Coll Cardiol* 1987; 10:568–575.

11. Spence PA, Peniston CM, David TE, et al: Toward a better understanding of the etiology of left ventricular dysfunction after mitral valve replacement. *Ann Thorac Surg* 1986; 4:363–371.

12. Goldman ME, Guarino T, Fuster V, et al: The necessity for tricuspid valve repair can be determined intraoperatively by two-dimensional echocardiography. *J Thorac Cardiovasc Surg* 1987; 94:542–550.

13. Mindich BP, Guarino T, Krenz H, et al: Aortic valve salvage utilizing high frequency vibratory debridement. *J Am Coll Cardiol* 1988; 11:3A.

14. Dubroff JM, Clark MB, Wong CY, et al: Left ventricular ejection fraction during cardiac surgery: A two-dimensional echocardiographic study. *Circulation* 1983; 68:95–103.

15. Topol EJ, Weiss JL, Guzman PA, et al: Immediate improvement of dysfunctional myocardial segments after coronary revascularization: Detection by intraoperative transesophageal echocardiography. *J Am Coll Cardiol* 1984; 4:1123–1134.

16. Douglas PS, Reichek N, Franklin K, et al: Intraoperative assessment of left ventricular heterogeneity. *Am Heart J* 1986; 112:344–349.

17. Gewertz BL, Kremser PC, Zarins CK, et al: Transesophageal echocardiographic monitoring of myocardial ischemia during vascular surgery. *J Vasc Surg* 1987; 5:607–613.

18. Roizen MF, Beaupre PN, Alpert RA, et al: Monitoring with two-dimensional transesophageal echocardiography: Comparison of myocardial function in patients undergoing supraceliac, suprarenal-infraceliac, or infrarenal aortic occlusion. *J Vasc Surg* 1984; 1:300–305.

19. Kyo S, Takamoto S, Matsumura M, et al: Immediate and early postoperative evaluation of results of cardiac surgery by transesophageal two-dimensional Doppler echocardiography. *Circulation* 1987; 76:VII3–VII21.

20. Smith JS, Cahalan MK, Benefiel DJ, et al: Intraoperative detection of myocardial ischemia in high-risk patients: Electrocardiography versus two-dimensional transesophageal echocardiography. *Circulation* 1985; 72:1015–1021.
21. Stewart WJ, Schiavone WA, Salcedo EE, et al: Intraoperative Doppler echocardiography in hypertrophic cardiomyopathy: Correlations with the obstructive gradient. *J Am Coll Cardiol* 1987; 10:327–335.
22. Sahn DJ, Copeland JG, Temkin LP, et al: Anatomic-ultrasound correlations for intraoperative open chest imaging of coronary artery atherosclerotic lesions in human beings. *J Am Coll Cardiol* 1984; 3:1169–1177.
23. Hiratzka LF, McPherson DD, Brandt B III, et al: The role of intraoperative high-frequency epicardial echocardiography during coronary artery revascularization. *Circulation* 1987; 76:V33–V38.
24. Goldman ME, Mindich BP: Intraoperative cardioplegic contrast echocardiography for assessing myocardial perfusion during open heart surgery. *J Am Coll Cardiol* 1984; 4:1029–1034.
25. Takamoto S, Kyo S, Adachi H, et al: Intraoperative color flow mapping by real-time two-dimensional Doppler echocardiography for evaluation of valvular and congenital heart disease and vascular disease. *J Thorac Cardiovasc Surg* 1985; 90:802–812.
26. Gussenhoven EJ, van Herwerden LA, Roelandt J, et al: Intraoperative two-dimensional echocardiography in congenital heart disease. *J Am Coll Cardiol* 1987; 9:565–572.
27. Hagler DJ, Tajik AJ, Seward JB, et al: Intraoperative two-dimensional Doppler echocardiography: A preliminary study for congenital heart disease. *J Thorac Cardiovasc Surg* 1988; 95:516–522.
28. Mora F, Mindich BP, Guarino T, et al: Improved surgical approach to cardiac tumors with intraoperative two-dimensional echocardiography. *Chest* 1987; 91:141–144.
29. Omoto R, Takamoto S, Kyo S, et al: The use of two-dimensional color Doppler sonography during the surgical management of aortic dissection. *World J Surg* 1987; 11:604–609.
30. Goldman ME, Guarino T, Mindich BP: Localization of aortic dissection intimal flap by intraoperative two-dimensional echocardiography. *J Am Coll Cardiol* 1985; 6:1155–1159.

Index